RECIPES & REMEDIES

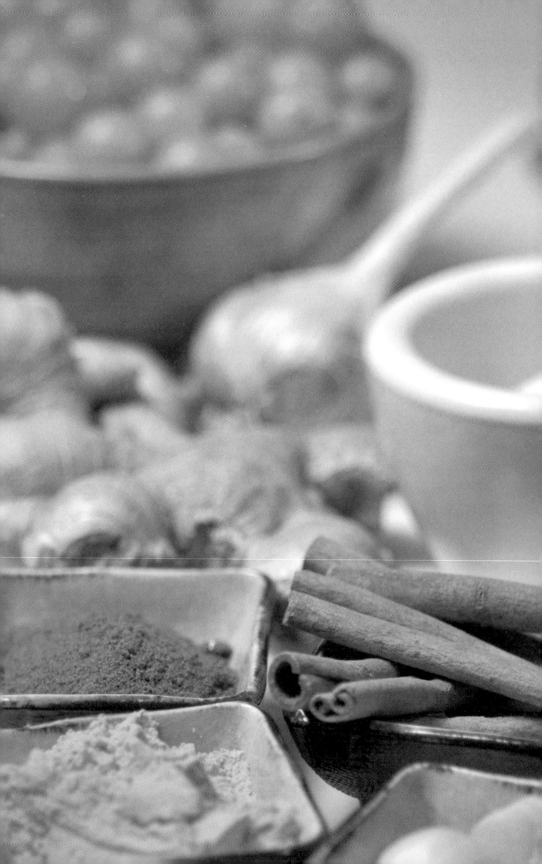

Recipes & Remedies

FROM THE PEOPLE'S PHARMACY

By Joe & Terry Graedon

ISBN 978 0615 40430 1

··· CONTENTS ···

RECIPES & REMEDIES FOR MANAGING COMMON CONDITIONS

TWO WEEKS OF HEALTHY & DELICIOUS MEALS & RECIPES

··· LIST OF REMEDIES ···

··· LIST OF RECIPES ···

BREAKFAST

MAIN DISHES

SIDE DISHES

DESSERTS

··· ACKNOWLEDGMENTS ···

Writing a book is often a solitary exercise. We are fortunate in that we write together, so it is not quite such an isolating experience. Nevertheless, creating a book from scratch is usually a bit lonely. This book was different. For one thing, the person who did all the heavy lifting was our daughter Alena. She is really the third author of this book, which could never have been completed without her extraordinary assistance. She contacted all our contributors, tested many of the recipes and created the glue that holds everything together. We are incredibly grateful.

We are so fortunate to have developed close relationships with many of the guests we interview on the radio. These are amazing people who graciously share their knowledge with our listeners. Now they are sharing their favorite recipes with you. These are people who understand the importance of food and nutrition for good health.

We owe a special debt of gratitude to Kristy Spencer, who came up with the original idea for the book *Favorite Foods from The People's Pharmacy: Mother Nature's Medicine*. While she and Joe were watching her husband Steve play a semi-finals tennis match with another friend, Keith Sipe, she suggested a book about food for good health. A year later she expanded on the original concept (again at the tennis courts) and proposed the idea for this book, specific recipes and remedies. We owe Keith Sipe a big thank you for helping us navigate the logistics of publishing. He also plays a mean game of tennis!

Jennifer Hill designed the book. Andrew Buchanan took the cover photo and all of the other photographs that appear throughout this book. Lyn Siegel helps make sure the books get to their intended recipients. We also want to thank public radio listeners and station personnel who help keep *The People's Pharmacy* show on the air every week.

Special thanks to all the following people who contributed their tasty recipes:

Sophie Barrett & Susannah Smith
Jeffrey Blumberg, PhD
Christopher Gardner, PhD
Alan Greene, MD
Cheryl Greene
Kit Gruelle
Mark Liponis, MD
Tieraona Low Dog, MD
David Mathis, MD, FAAFP, ABHM, D.Ay
Debbie Mathis, MA, D.Ay
Sally Fallon Morell
Michael Ozner, MD, FACC, FAHA
Helen Rasmussen, PhD, RD, FADA
Eric Westman, MD, MHS
Walter C. Willett, MD, Dr PH
Gail Pettiford Willett, RN
Steven Zeisel, MD, PhD
Susan Zeisel, EdD

··· NOTE TO THE READER ···

The recipes and remedies recommended in this book are not meant to be a substitute for proper diagnosis and appropriate medical treatment. Any health problems that do not get better promptly or get worse should be evaluated and treated by an appropriate clinician. Readers should always consult their own health care providers about any symptoms that may require diagnosis or medical attention.

Foods and dietary supplements do not agree with everyone. Some people may be allergic to certain foods or ingredients and must use good common sense in evaluating and responding to such reactions. If you suspect that you are or someone you care for is experiencing an adverse reaction to a food, dietary supplement, or home remedy, please consult a knowledgeable health professional immediately.

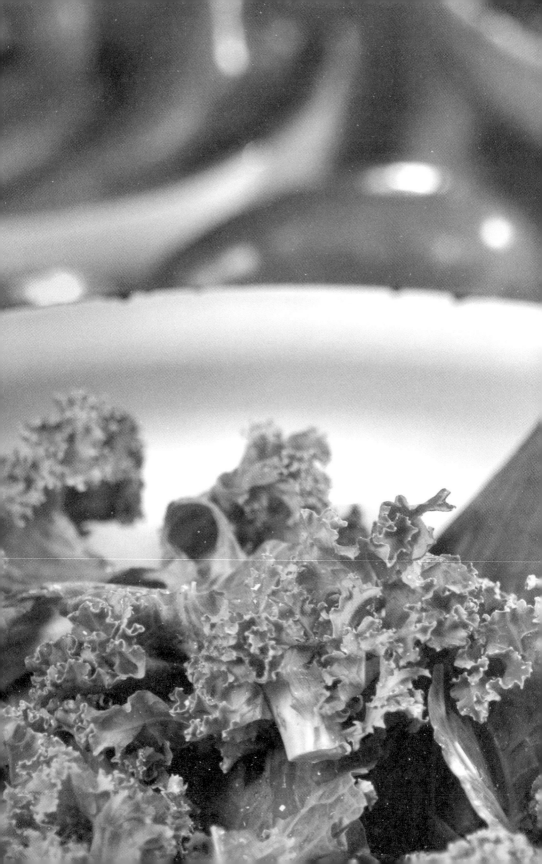

··· INTRODUCTION ···

We have been interested in using food as medicine for decades. When a reader suggested the idea of a book discussing our favorite foods for health and pulling together all the information we had about using specific foods for specific ailments, we were a bit skeptical at first. On reflection, though, we realized that food is a critical component of everything we do at The People's Pharmacy, whether on the radio, in the newspaper column or in books. Our most popular home remedies tend to involve food: gin-soaked raisins or Certo in grape juice for arthritis, cherries for gout, or lemon juice against kidney stones. So we concluded that it was a great idea. When we started collecting food remedies and information, we were impressed to discover how much scientific research had been done recently on the medicinal uses of food. But we never could have imagined the overwhelming response to *Favorite Foods from The People's Pharmacy*, which we published in 2009.

Favorite Foods took a two-pronged approach to the idea of using food as medicine: first, it listed our favorite foods, beverages, and supplements, and explained how they could be used to treat or prevent specific medical conditions, such as using beet juice for high blood pressure. Second, it outlined three popular diets: DASH (Dietary Approaches to Stop Hypertension), low-carbohydrate, and Mediterranean, and recommended using the food we eat as medicine in a more general, holistic way—by adopting a healthy diet to achieve health.

We were surprised and gratified by the outpouring of interest in *Favorite Foods*, but we continued to hear from listeners and readers who had questions about how to put the second part of that approach into practice. We all talk about eating healthy food, but how do we do it?

The same reader who suggested *Favorite Foods* encouraged us to get specific. She wanted recipes and meal plans. We thought other readers would appreciate those, too. So we contacted some of our favorite guests from *The People's Pharmacy* radio show—leading national experts in nutrition and health—and we asked them to send us some of their favorite healthful recipes. We then chose from that select group, and we added some of our own favorite recipes to the mix, as we also love to cook—and eat!

The experts we consulted represent a diversity of opinions about the best ways to use food to achieve optimal health. We've solicited recipes from specialists in Ayurvedic medicine, vegetarians, omnivores, locavores, proponents of the Mediterranean Diet, those who follow a low-carbohydrate method, food scientists, and others. Sometimes their positions diverge, but there are also many places where they overlap. Everyone, for instance, advocates integrating as many fresh, seasonal vegetables as possible. And while we see great value in all of their different approaches, we are not strict adherents to any one diet. We tend to mix things up a bit in our kitchen, and we've done so here.

We also integrated recipes for a variety of remedies, devoting the first section of this book to describing which remedy-recipes to use for managing a number of common health conditions. All of the food recipes are organized into meal plans for two weeks of delicious and healthful eating, arranged seasonally: one week for spring and summer meals, one for fall and winter. Because we think that eating for health involves eating as many fresh vegetables and fruits as possible, we wanted to be sure to recommend recipes for foods during the times of year that they're most readily available. The result is what you hold in your hands. This is what healthy eating looks like to us. We hope some of these recipes will become your favorites, too.

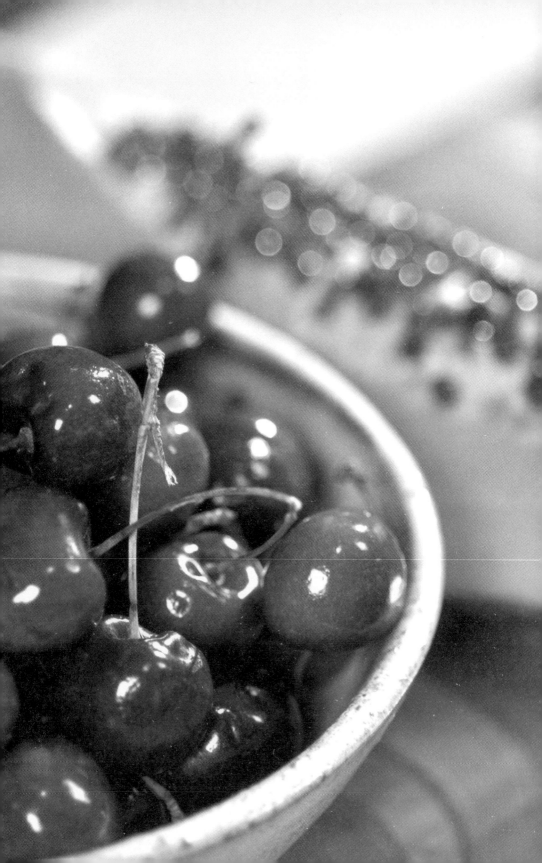

Recipes & Remedies

FOR MANAGING
COMMON CONDITIONS

··· MANAGING BLOOD SUGAR ···

Maintaining safe blood sugar levels is obviously a very serious undertaking. Regular blood sugar tests and the vigilant care of a physician are absolutely essential for anyone with diabetes. No one should ever change or discontinue a course of medication or treatment without her doctor's careful supervision.

But even those of us who are not diabetic could benefit from keeping our blood sugar in a healthy range and not letting our levels spike too much or too often. Below are a few simple recipes that may help reduce insulin resistance.

Bitter Melon Stir Fry (see page 112)

True to its name, bitter melon is a very astringent gourd that is much more common in other parts of the world (for example India and China) than it is in the U.S. It's an acquired taste for many, but several studies have shown that it can be effective in helping to manage blood sugar levels (see, i.e., Nerurkar, et al, 2010), and different methods of preparation can help to remove the bitter taste.

Cinnamon Coffee

Cinnamon has also been shown to lower blood glucose (Solomon and Blannin, 2009). One danger of daily cinnamon ingestion, however, is that the compound coumarin, which sometimes occurs in cassia cinnamon, can inflame the liver in large doses. Unlike the active compounds in cinnamon that lower blood sugar, coumarin isn't water soluble. As a result, one potential fix that we have tried is to add cinnamon to our coffee grounds in the morning, and then to filter them both through a paper filter. You will still want to be sure to check your liver enzymes regularly at the doctor, however, if you are considering adding cinnamon to your daily diet.

4 scoops of freshly ground coffee beans
½ teaspoon of ground cinnamon

Place grounds and cinnamon in a paper filter. Pour boiling water over the mixture and let the coffee brew through to a waiting mug. This should be plenty for two strong cups.

Cinnamon-Almond Oatmeal (see page 105)

Some research indicates that almonds may also help to prevent spikes in blood sugar, especially when eaten with simple carbohydrates like white bread (Josse, et al, 2007). The recipe in this book shouldn't be eaten every day—there is a potential danger of liver damage from the coumarin that can sometimes be found in cinnamon, and there also may be too many calories in the almonds unless adjustments are made to other parts of your diet. But it can certainly be enjoyed as part of a healthy, balanced menu plan.

Fenugreek Seed Tea

Some exciting animal studies indicate that fenugreek may be very useful as a supplementary alternative treatment for those with diabetes (Uemura, et al, 2010). More research in humans is needed, but in the meantime, this recipe for fenugreek tea certainly can't hurt. It can be consumed hot or cold. We recommended drinking two to three glasses per day.

> 1 teaspoon fenugreek seeds
> 8 ounces water
> Lemon and non-calorie sweetener to taste

Place fenugreek seeds in a mug, and pour boiling water over them. Allow the seeds to steep for 10 to 15 minutes. Strain out the seeds. Add lemon and non-calorie sweetener to taste, and either enjoy the beverage hot, or store it in the refrigerator to drink later.

Mustard and Vinegar Dressing

Vinegar has been proven to have positive effects on blood glucose (Johnston, et al, 2009), and we have heard from at least one diabetic reader that mustard may have a similar result. One easy and delicious way to consume both at once is in this superb homemade vinaigrette, which we eat on salad or coleslaw almost daily. The recipe below makes enough for one salad that two people can enjoy.

> ½ tablespoon olive oil
> ½ to 1 whole garlic clove, passed through a press
> 1 tablespoon mustard

1 tablespoon vinegar of your choosing
Salt and pepper to taste

In a small bowl, combine the olive oil, garlic, salt, pepper, and mustard. Whisk with a fork until the mixture is thick (about the consistency of aioli). Then add the vinegar, and whisk again until evenly combined. Use right away.

Q *I am a nurse, and one of my patients has a success story that may interest you. His presurgical tests showed an HbA_{1c} above 8, indicating that his blood sugar had been above normal for months. He decided to start taking a cinnamon supplement.*

  When I saw him two months later, his HbA_{1c} was 6.0. Wow! He's also been taking a teaspoon of yellow mustard, which contains vinegar and turmeric, after every meal. It muddies the research, but it has been good for him.

A Thanks so much for sharing this story. HbA_{1c} is a blood test that reveals long-term blood sugar control. Keeping the level below 7 is considered desirable.

  Not everyone benefits from cinnamon, but we have heard from readers that a supplement can be helpful. There is even some research to support this approach (*Journal of Diabetes Science and Technology*, May, 2010). Both vinegar and turmeric can help reduce the rise in blood sugar after eating, so we're not surprised that mustard might be beneficial too.

Wheat Berry Salad (see page 154)

Jeffrey Blumberg, PhD and Helen Rasmussen, PhD, RD, FADA specifically designed their wheat berry salad to have a low glycemic index. As they note, "Foods with a lower glycemic index produce smaller increases in blood glucose and insulin than those with a high glycemic index." That makes them better for those looking to manage their blood sugar.

··· REFERENCES ···

Johnston, C. S., White, A. M., and Kent, S. M. "Preliminary evidence that regular vinegar ingestion favorably influences hemoglobin A1c values in individuals with type 2 diabetes mellitus." *Diabetes Research and Clinical Practice* 2009; 84(2): e15- e17.

Josse, A.R., et al. "Almonds and postprandial glycemia—a dose-response study." *Metabolism* 2007; 56(3): 400-404.

Nerurkar, P.V., Lee, Y.K., and Nerurkar, V.R. "*Momordica charantia* (bitter melon) inhibits primary human adipocyte differentiation by modulating adipogenic genes." BMC *Complement Altern Med.* 2010; 10(1):34. [Epub ahead of print]

Solomon, T. P., and Blannin, A. K. "Changes in glucose tolerance and insulin sensitivity following 2 weeks of daily cinnamon ingestion in healthy humans." *European Journal of Applied Physiology* 2009; 105(6):969-976.

Uemura, T., et al. "Diosgenin present in fenugreek improves glucose metabolism by promoting adipocyte differentiation and inhibiting inflammation in adipose tissues." *Mol Nutr Food Res.* 2010. [Epub ahead of print]

··· FIGHTING CANCER ···

Over the past several years, we have become convinced that being conscientious about the kinds of foods we eat is one of the single most important ways we can mitigate our risk for developing cancer. There are of course many risk factors that are out of our control—genetics and exposure to environmental toxins chief among them. There are also many other things that we can do to better our odds for staying healthy, including getting regular exercise, trying to avoid stress, and maintaining healthy social connections. But food is at the center of all of our lives. And depending on what we eat, it may help to increase and improve the quality of our lives for years to come.

One of the experts responsible for changing our perception about the role of diet in preventing cancer is David Servan-Schreiber, M.D., Ph.D. Dr. Servan-Schreiber is a clinical professor of psychiatry, a neuroscientist, and a brain cancer survivor. His brain cancer was discovered in a most unusual way: while helping to run a laboratory, he offered to stand in to receive a MRI one day when a volunteer study subject did not show up. His colleagues noticed an abnormality on the scan that turned out to be a tumor. After surgery and chemotherapy, his oncologists told him that he was free to go home and enjoy his life as normal. He asked them what he could do to prevent the cancer from recurring, but they shrugged off the question.

It wasn't until several years later, when the cancer returned and he had to go undergo radiation and a second course of chemotherapy, that Dr. Servan-Schreiber decided to change his life radically. Diet was at the center of that change. Dr. Servan-Schreiber gravitated toward the French concept of the body's internal "terrain," and on the healthy functioning of the body as a whole system. We strongly recommend Dr. Servan-Schreiber's book to anyone interested in this idea. It's called *Anticancer: A New Way of Life.*

Dr. Servan-Schreiber has convinced us that certain foods—specifically starches, refined sugars, white flour, and other simple carbohydrates—can cause inflammation and lead to cancer cell growth. A small Italian study reinforces the results of prior research on pancreatic cancer and diet. The investigators questioned 326 people with pancreatic cancer about their diet and lifestyle. Each patient was matched to two healthy adults who answered the same questions. The research team found that a third of the people, those who ate the most sugary foods, were 78 percent more likely than those in the lowest third to have pancreatic cancer. The worst offenders were sweet foods that raise blood sugar quickly, like jam, candy, honey and sugar. There was no link with diabetes or obesity. The absolute risk for any individual is still low, since pancreatic cancer is relatively rare. But together with earlier research showing a link between sugary drinks and pancreatic cancer, this study suggests that regular consumption of sweets may increase the risk of this rare but deadly disease. [Rossi, et al, 2010]

Dr. Servan-Schreiber thinks that some foods have special cancer-fighting properties. After considering his research and doing some investigating of our own, we've developed a list of top cancer-fighting foods (and one beverage). We think that these foods are important not only for reducing one's risk of developing cancer, but also for promoting overall good health. Listed below are our favorite cancer-fighting foods in order of most to least powerful, along with recipe ideas for many of them.

··· TOP ANTICANCER FOODS ···

Garlic
   Roasted Garlic (see page 151)
Leeks
   Leek and Sweet Onion Frittata (see page 129)
Brussels Sprouts
   Roasted Brussels Sprouts (see page 150)
Scallions
   Scallions appear in many recipes throughout these pages. See, for instance, *Quinoa Radish Salad* on page 140; *Shrimp & Grits* on page 111; *Grilled Tofu & Avocado Salad with Blood Orange Vinaigrette* on page 123; and *Bitter Melon Stir Fry* on page 112.
Cabbage
   Cancer-Fighting Cabbage Curry (see page 115)
   Coleslaw with Mint (see page 145)
Beets
   Beet Juice Smoothie (see page 34)
   Farmer's Market Saag (see page 146)
Broccoli
   Broccoli and Garlic Stir Fry (see page 49)
   Penne with Broccoli and Sundried Tomatoes (see page 136)
Cauliflower
   Cauliflower and Red Pepper Quiche (see page 118)
Onions
   Onions appear in recipes throughout this book.

Kale
  Kale Chips (see page 148)
  Farmer's Market Saag (see page 146)
Spinach
  Poached Eggs with Spinach (see page 110)
Asparagus
  Poached Eggs and Asparagus (see page 138)
Green Tea*

  *ONE CAVEAT ON GREEN TEA: people being treated for
  multiple myeloma with a drug called bortezomib should
  avoid it. One of the compounds in green tea, epigallocate-
  chin-3-gallate, or EGCG, can prevent bortezomib from killing
  cancer (Golden, et al, 2009). Indeed, we think it would
  probably be wise for anyone on chemotherapy to check with
  her oncologist before adding green tea to her daily regimen.
Turnips
  Farmer's Market Saag (see page 146)
Squash
  Israeli Couscous with Roasted Summer Vegetables & Nuts
  (see page 128)
  Butternut Squash and Apple Soup (see page 113)
Celery
  Curry Soup (see page 119)
Radishes
  Fish Tacos with Radish and Lime (see page 120)
  Quinoa amd Radish Salad (see page 140)
Eggplant
  Baba Ganoush (see *Veggie Dips*, page 153)
Bok Choy
Carrots
  Lentil and Roasted Bell Pepper Salad (see page 133)

Along with the foods listed above, there are also a few foods,
another beverage, and a spice that may be beneficial in targeting

specific cancers. Coffee, for instance, which is surprisingly rich in antioxidants, has been shown to lower the risk for cancers of the mouth, throat, and esophagus (Naganuma, et al, 2008), colon (Je et al, 2009), kidneys (Lee et al, 2007), liver (Montella et al, 2007), skin (Kerzendorfer, et al, 2009; Heffernan, et al, 2009), and endometrium (McCann, et al, 2009). If you add a bit of cinnamon to the grounds of your morning cup of drip coffee, you may also help reduce your insulin resistance. (See *Cinnamon Coffee*, page 8.)

In pre-clinical trials with animals, pomegranates have been shown to prevent the growth of breast, prostate, colon, and lung cancer cells when grown in the laboratory. Some initial results have also shown encouraging outcomes in a prostate cancer clinical trial (Adhami, et al, 2009). We are huge fans of pomegranates and try to incorporate them into our diet whenever possible. One way is in the form of juice, like in *Joe's Brain-Boosting Smoothie* (see page 107).

Two comestibles that may qualify more as spices than foods are hot peppers and turmeric. Both contain ingredients that appear to have significant anti-cancer properties. In the case of hot peppers, the ingredient is capsaicin, which is what makes hot peppers hot. And in turmeric, the vital ingredient is curcumin. Literally hundreds of studies have demonstrated the anticancer properties of curcumin, and new research has recently been undertaken suggesting that capsaicin may also ward off a range of cancers (Aggarwal, et al, 2008; Kuramori, et al, 2009; Yang, et al, 2009).

We're big proponents of both seasonings, and we try to add them to as many dishes as we can. For recipes containing hot peppers, see our *Pescado al Cilantro* (page 137); and for turmeric-laced dishes, see: *Anti-Inflammatory Curcumin Scramble* (page 103), *Curry Soup* (page 119), *Curried Sweet Potato Fries* (page 145), and *Cancer-Fighting Cabbage Curry* (page 115).

ONE IMPORTANT CAUTION: those taking the blood-thinner warfarin (Coumadin) should avoid curcumin, since it may increase the risk of bleeding.

··· REFERENCES ···

Adhami, V.M., Khan, N., and Mukhtar, H. "Cancer chemoprevention by pomegranate: laboratory and clinical evidence." *Nutrition and Cancer* 2009; 61(6):811-5.

Aggarwal, B. B., et al. "Potential of spice-derived phytochemicals for cancer prevention." *Planta Medica* 2008;74(13):1560-1569.

Golden, E. B., Lam, P. Y., et al. "Green tea polyphenols block the anti-cancer effects of bortezomib and other boronic acid-based proteasome inhibitors." *Blood* 2009; 113(23):5927-5937.

Heffernan, Timothy P., Kawasumi, Masaoki, et al. "ATR–Chk1 pathway inhibition promotes apoptosis after UV treatment in primary human keratinocytes: Potential basis for the UV protective effects of caffeine." *Journal of Investigative Dermatology* 2009; 129:1805-1815.

Je, Youjin, Liu, Wei, et al. "Coffee consumption and risk of colorectal cancer: A systematic review and meta-analysis of prospective cohort studies. *International Journal of Cancer* 2009; 124(7):1662-1668.

Kerzendorfer, Claudia, and O'Driscoll, Mark. "UVB and caffeine: inhibiting the DNA damage response to protect against the adverse effects of UVB." *Journal of Investigative Dermatology* 2009; 129:1611-1613.

Kuramori, C., et al. "Capsaicin binds to prohibitin 2 and displaces it from the mitochondria to the nucleus." *Biochemical and Biophysical Research Communications* 2009; 379(2):519-525.

Lee, Jung Eun, Hunter, David J., et al. "Intakes of coffee, tea, milk, soda and juice and renal cell cancer in a pooled analysis of 13 prospective studies." *International Journal of Cancer* 2007; 121(10):2246-2253.

McCann, Susan E., Yeh, Michael, et al. "Higher regular coffee and tea consumption is associated with reduced endometrial cancer risk." *International Journal of Cancer* 2009; 124(7):1650-1653.

Montella, Maurizio, Polesel, Jerry, et al. "Coffee and tea consumption and risk of hepatocellular carcinoma in Italy." *International Journal of Cancer* 2007; 120(7):1555-1559.

Naganuma, Toru, Kuriyama, Shinichi, et al. "Coffee consumption and the risk of oral, pharyngeal, and esophageal cancers in Japan: The Miyagi Cohort Study." *American Journal of Epidemiology* 2008; 168:1425-1432.

Rossi, Marta, Lipworth, Loren, et al. "Dietary glycemic index and glycemic load and risk of pancreatic cancer: a case-control study." *Ann. Epidemiol.* 2010; 20(6):460-465.

Servan-Schreiber, David *Anti-Cancer: A New Way of Life.* (New York: Viking, 2008).

Yang, K. M., et al "Capsaicin induces apoptosis by generating reactive oxygen species and disrupting mitochondrial transmembrane potential in human colon cancer cell lines." *Cellular and Molecular Biology Letters* 2009; 14(3):497-510.

··· LOWERING CHOLESTEROL ···

Cholesterol-lowering medications are among the most widely prescribed drugs in the world. And while they're quite effective at doing what they were designed to do, i.e. lower cholesterol, it's less clear that these results necessarily translate into fewer deaths (Ray, et al, 2010). On top of that, statin medications are expensive, and for many people, they can cause quite unpleasant side effects: muscle and nerve pain, weakness, cognitive impairment, and short-term memory loss.

We don't mean to imply that statins aren't useful for some people. But they may be overprescribed. There are lots of ways in which people can lower their bad LDL cholesterol and triglycerides and raise their good HDL cholesterol without a prescription. It's been well established that fish oil is very good at lowering bad cholesterol and boosting good cholesterol, as are nuts like walnuts and almonds. Oatmeal and oat bran can also lower total cholesterol, and an interesting animal study showed that the ingredient cinnamate in cinnamon brought cholesterol and triglyceride levels down in rats even better than the drug lovastatin did (Lee, et al, 2003).

"I used to have very high total cholesterol (in the 350 range), and reduced it over time to a total cholesterol level of 185 (including HDL in 65 to 70 range) strictly through diet and exercise.

I consume all of the foods and beverages that are supposed to be good for reducing cholesterol (olive oil, fish oil, oatmeal, Concord grape juice, pomegranate juice, walnuts, dark chocolate, etc.). I don't do so only to lower my cholesterol but as a part of a healthy, vegetarian diet (supplemented with fish oil).

For me, it began with a paradigm switch: I went from eating what I liked and wanted to eat to eating what my body wanted me to eat. Once I gained some knowledge and began asking that question—what does my body want me to eat?—my health improved immediately and has continued to improve over the past decade. I've gone from 315 pounds to 190 pounds and to a BMI of 24.

Vinegar also seems to bring total cholesterol and triglycerides down in rats (Fushimi, et al, 2006).

Avoiding certain foods is another good way to improve cholesterol. A recent study showed that a low-carbohydrate diet was better at lowering triglycerides and raising good cholesterol than a standard low-fat diet was (Shai, et al, 2008).

Listed below are some of our favorite recipes for balancing good and bad cholesterol, along with the page numbers where you can find them in this book.

Oatmeal
    Cholesterol-Combating Oatmeal
    (see page 104)
    Cinnamon-Almond Oatmeal
    (see page 105)
Vinegar
    Mustard and Vinegar Dressing
    (see page 9)

··· REFERENCES ···

Fushimi, T., Suruga, K., et al. "Dietary acetic acid reduces serum cholesterol and triacylglycerols in rats fed a cholesterol-rich diet." *British Journal of Nutrition* 2006; 95(5):916-24.

Lee, J. S., Jeon, S. M., et al. "Cinnamate supplementation enhances hepatic lipid metabolism and antioxidant defense systems in high cholesterol-fed rats." *Journal of Medicinal Food* 2003; 6(3):183-91.

Ray, Kausik K., Seshasai, Sreenivasa Rao Kondapally, et al. "Statins and All-Cause Mortality in High-Risk Primary Prevention: A Meta-analysis of 11 Randomized Controlled Trials Involving 65,229 Participants." *Archives of Internal Medicine* 2010; 170(12):1024-1031.

Shai, I., Schwarzfuchs, D., et al. "Weight loss with a low-carbohydrate, Mediterranean, or low-fat diet." *New England Journal of Medicine* 2008; 359(3): 229-41.

I don't take any prescription drugs and would only ever do so as a last resort. If I tried all the healthy, natural alternatives and nothing worked, then I'd give pharmaceuticals a try. I truly believe that if people follow commonsense guidelines on diet and exercise, then high cholesterol, type II diabetes, and all related maladies would mostly disappear.

The writer Michael Pollan's advice, 'Eat food, not too much, mostly plants,' is a good starting point. Once people start doing the basics, they see that plant-based foods work such miracles that they continually gravitate more in that direction."

··· FIGHTING COLDS AND COUGHS ···

W e all know what we're supposed to do to try to keep from getting sick: wash our hands; get plenty of rest, especially when we feel we're coming down with something; and stay bundled up (Johnson et al, 2005). But we've long heard that once you're sick, you're stuck. That really there's nothing you can do but ride the illness out.

This is true to a certain extent: the thing that's most effective against a cold is time—but maybe also thyme. Germans, especially well-educated women, are quick to administer herbal medicine to their children (Hümer, et al, 2010). That may explain why a study was conducted in Germany several years ago to determine whether or not a thyme-primrose mixture would help ease the symptoms of acute bronchitis. In the study, which was double-blind and placebo-controlled, the subjects were adults. And after 11 days of evaluation, researchers found that the combination worked significantly better than placebo (Kemmerich, 2007). It was also safe and well tolerated. We've gathered many stories from listeners and readers over the years who have benefited from a variety of thyme-infused broths and teas for easing their coughs, and we've put together quite a collection of recipes. You'll find several below.

Another old cold standby is chicken soup. It turns out there's a reason. Chicken soup's not just good for the soul: it's also good for colds. Many years ago, researchers at Mt. Sinai Medical Center in Miami did a study to see whether hot water, cold water, or chicken soup was better at getting mucus going. The winner? Chicken soup, by a nose (Saketkhoo, et al, 1978). Another study indicated that eating chicken soup can help reduce the inflammation that's brought about by immune-system cells called neutrophils (Rennard, 2000). And there was also an evidence-based review several years ago demonstrating that chicken soup most likely helps alleviate flu symptoms (Jefferson, 2002). You'll find several recipes below featuring this illustrious bird.

Chicken Adobo (see page 118)

Coconut Chicken Soup
Contributed by Sally Fallon Morell

1 quart homemade chicken broth
1 can (14 ounces) whole coconut milk
The juice of one lemon
1 tablespoon grated fresh ginger
1 teaspoon sea salt
A pinch of red pepper flakes

To prepare the homemade chicken broth: place the leftover carcass of a chicken (bones, skin, and any additional meat) in a large pot, and cover with cold water. Add salt and pepper. Bring water to a boil, then immediately reduce heat to a low simmer. Cook uncovered for several hours, occasionally skimming the foam from the surface of the broth. Remove the bones and strain the broth.

To prepare the soup: combine all ingredients in a large saucepan. Stir together, and bring to a simmer. Makes four servings.

Sally Fallon Morell has told us: "This is great for colds and the flu."

Helen Graedon's Chicken Soup

I large stewing hen and a few additional backs and wings
I large onion, peeled and chopped
2 to 3 carrots, peeled and sliced
Several parsnips, peeled and chopped
Fresh parsley
5 to 6 bay leaves
6 cloves of garlic, peeled
Salt and pepper to taste
I cup fresh or frozen peas
½ cup noodles or rice

Place the stewing hen, backs and wings in a pot. Cover with water and top with two inches more. Add the onions, carrots, parsnip, parsley, bay leaves, garlic, pepper and salt. Simmer for about two hours, then strain out the chicken, vegetables and spices. Remove the meat of the chicken from the bones (careful—it will be hot!), and add it back to the soup with peas, noodles or rice. Refrigerating the broth overnight makes it easy to skim the excess fat off the top.

Ginger Tea (see page 56)

Ginger & Thyme Broth

1 cube of chicken bouillon
1 cup hot water
1 teaspoon fresh ginger, peeled and grated
½ teaspoon dried time, or 1 teaspoon fresh time

Dissolve the cube of bouillon in the hot water. Add the ginger and thyme. Steep the mixture for four or five minutes and then pour it through a strainer into a clean mug and sip.

Q *For two consecutive years after a prolonged, forceful cough that lasted one or two months, I totally lost my voice. My* ENT *doctor diagnosed me with chronic laryngitis and prescribed medication and lozenges. They offered no relief, though.*

Then I was told by the old women from our home place, the Philippines, to avoid cold drinks and to take "salabat." That's ginger tea in our dialect. My voice returned. Ginger tea is also good for sore throat and hoarse voice.

A Ginger has a long history in treating nausea, vomiting, flatulence and other digestive disorders. It has also been used for congestion, cough and bronchitis. Thanks for letting us know how well it worked for your laryngitis.

Another reader had a great experience with ginger for a persistent cough: "Ginger is amazing! I had a really dry cough that went on for three weeks. I tried antibiotics, mucolytics, gargles and anesthetic lozenges but they didn't work. Then my father suggested that I chop some raw ginger root, chew the pieces like candy and suck the juice out of them. I tried it and the following day, my cough was gone."

Hot Toddy

1 teaspoon sugar
8 ounces boiling water
1 tablespoon lemon juice
1 shot (about 1½ ounces) rum

Put the sugar in the bottom of a mug or heat-safe glass. Add the hot water, lemon juice, and rum. Stir vigorously. Stay home, sip, and relax.

T's Immuno-Tea
Contributed by Tieraona Low Dog, MD

1 ounce astragalus root, dried and sliced
1 ounce schizandra fruit, dried
1 ounce rose hips, dried
½ ounce eleuthero root, dried and sliced
Honey and lemon to taste

Mix herbs together and store in a jar. Keep in a dark place.

To prepare: put one tablespoon herb mixture into two cups water, bring to a boil, and simmer, covered, for 15 minutes. Strain. Add honey and lemon to taste.

Dr. Low Dog recommends: "Drink half a cup two to three times per day during the cold and flu season."

Thyme Cough Syrup
Contributed by Tieraona Low Dog, MD

1 cup water
2 tablespoons dried thyme (or 4 tablespoons fresh)
1 teaspoon lemon juice
½ cup organic honey

Pour one cup near-boiling water over thyme and steep for 10 minutes. Strain. Add honey and lemon juice. Refrigerate for up to one week. For children 18 months and older: take one tablespoon as needed.

For those who don't like the flavor of thyme, substitute fennel seed. Simmer the seeds gently on low heat for 15 minutes, then strain.

Thyme Tea

½ teaspoon dried thyme
8 ounces boiling water

Pour the boiling water over the thyme and allow to steep for five or six minutes. Strain the leaves out through a strainer and sweeten to taste.

··· REFERENCES ···

Hümer, M., Scheller, G., et al. ["Use of herbal medicine in German children — prevalence, indications and motivation."Article in German] *Dtsch Med Wochenschr.* 2010; 135(19):959-64. Epub 2010 May 5.

Jefferson, T. "Advances in the diagnosis and management of influenza." *Current Infectious Disease Reports* 2002; 4(3):206-210.

Johnson, C., and Eccles, R. "Acute cooling of the feet and the onset of common cold symptoms." *Family Practice* 2005; 22(6):608-13.

Kemmerich, B. "Evaluation of efficacy and tolerability of a fixed combination of dry extracts of thyme herb and primrose root in adults suffering from acute bronchitis with productive cough. A prospective, double-blind, placebo-controlled multicentre clinical trial." *Arzneimittelforschung.* 2007; 57(9):607-15.

Rennard, B. A., Ertle, R. D., et al. "Chicken soup inhibits neutrophil chemotaxis in vitro." *Chest* 2000; 118(10):1150-1155.

Saketkhoo, K., Januszkiewicz, A., and Sackner, M.A. "Effects of drinking hot water, cold water, and chicken soup on nasal mucus velocity and nasal airflow resistance." *Chest.* 1978; 74(4):408-10.

··· PREVENTING HYPERTENSION ···

There are lots of medications that successfully control high blood pressure. Some people benefit from diuretics while others get the most effective results from ACE inhibitors. If one anti-hypertensive doesn't work for you, there are dozens of others that you and your doctor can try. All of them, however, have the potential for side effects. Diuretics can cause magnesium and potassium deficiencies as well as sexual side effects, and ACE inhibitors have been known to give some people a constant, dry, hacking cough.

As we've said before and will say again, no one should ever alter any course of treatment without the care and guidance of a physician, particularly not with respect to something as serious as blood pressure. But if you're looking for a non-drug approach to getting your blood pressure under better control, there are many things you can try. A good place to start is with weight loss—losing even just a few pounds can make a big difference in blood pressure, and we hope that some of the healthful recipes in these pages may make this a little easier. Exercise is another good method for bringing those blood pressure numbers down. Learning to breathe more slowly, either through meditation or the help of a prescription RESPeRATE machine, is an additional technique many have found useful.

Diet can also play a big role in controlling hypertension. Reducing salt can help some people (He, et al, 2005). And the DASH (Dietary Approaches to Stop Hypertension) Diet has proven quite effective at lowering blood pressure (Al-Solaiman, et al, 2009; Appel, et al, 1997), especially when combined with exercise and weight loss (Blumenthal, et al, 2010). For more information on the DASH Diet, you can visit: http://dashdiet.org/ or http://www.nhlbi.nih. gov/health/public/heart/hbp/dash/new_dash.pdf. Or you can find out more from a book published by researchers involved in the original DASH study: The DASH* *Diet for Hypertension: Lower Your Blood Pressure in 14 Days—Without Drugs*, by Thomas Moore, MD, and his colleagues (New York: Free Press, 2001).

There are also some specific foods that seem to have a surprising effect on blood pressure. Below are some of the recipes we've gathered that utilize these foods.

Beet Juice Smoothie

An exciting study published a few years ago in the journal *Hypertension* showed that people who drank two cups of beet juice could lower their blood pressure by around 10 points (Webb, et al, 2008). Those results are similar to what most people get by taking blood pressure medications.

Needless to say, though, two cups is a lot of beet juice. If you're wondering where to find beet juice, it's possible to buy it at some health food stores or online. That could get expensive (although perhaps no more expensive than a prescription). If you have a juicer, you can also make your own.

If you're wondering what to *do* with two cups of beet juice, here is one suggestion:

2 cups beet juice
1 cup apple juice
1 cup carrot juice, or several carrots, peeled and chopped
2 tablespoons fresh ginger, peeled and grated
1 cup crushed ice
1 teaspoon fish oil
4 tablespoons whey powder

Puree all ingredients in a blender until smooth. You will probably need to scrape down the sides a few times. Pour into tall glasses or refrigerate for up to two days.

Q *I have been dealing with high blood pressure for years. When I am under stress my blood pressure goes up to around 150.*

My doctor has prescribed lots of different drugs with mixed results. Atenolol caused fatigue and depression. Amlodipine made me dizzy to the point I couldn't function. Lisinopril caused a horrible cough. Now I am on Diovan with no problems, but I read recently that drugs like this are linked with cancer.

I am ready to try a more natural approach. I heard that beets can lower blood pressure. How effective are they and what else might help?

A An article in *Lancet Oncology* (Sipahi, et al, 2010) has raised questions about the safety of drugs like Atacand, Diovan and Micardis. The investigators analyzed many scientific studies and concluded that such drugs "are associated with a modestly increased risk of new cancer occurrence." Drug regulators and clinicians don't know what to make of this new information.

An article published in the journal *Hypertension* (Kapil, et al, 2010) suggests that about 8.5 ounces of beet juice can significantly lower systolic blood pressure.

Three-Layer Mousse (see page 161)

Okay, so mousse may seem like a stretch for bringing blood pressure down. And we agree that it should be only an occasional treat, particularly for those who are trying to lose weight (a much more efficacious way to control hypertension than indulging in dessert). But there is growing evidence that flavanol-rich cocoa and dark chocolate may help bring down high blood pressure (see Buijsse, et al, 2010; Grassi, et al, 2010; Ried, et al, 2010, among other recent studies). Eating dark chocolate during pregnancy may even reduce the risk of preeclampsia for some women (Saftlas, 2010), although more research is needed.

The suggested daily "dose" is anywhere from 10 grams (about the size of a small Ghiradelli chocolate square) to 100 grams (the size of a Ritter Sport bar). But 100 grams of chocolate per day will make most people gain far too much weight to make the modest benefits worthwhile. We recommend going light on the dark chocolate—staying closer to the 10-gram end of the spectrum and making other caloric adjustments in your diet as needed to make sure you don't tip the scales. One preliminary study supports these recommendations, finding that people benefited from a decrease in blood pressure whether they ate a small or large amount of chocolate—and that those who ate more gained more (Desch, et al, 2010).

We have to confess that we're thrilled by these data, as we love dark chocolate. And whether consumed on its own or in recipes like our *Three-Layer Mousse* or *Poached Pears with Bittersweet Cocoa Sauce* (see page TK), dark chocolate is a far more healthful dessert than many you might find in the bakery aisle.

Eggplant Water

We've heard from several readers who swear by "eggplant water" to lower their blood pressure. No scientific evidence supports these readers' findings, but there is at least one study suggesting that compounds in eggplant may work in a way similar to ACE inhibitors and may also help with insulin resistance (Kwon et al, 2008).

6 thin slices of raw eggplant
2 quarts water

Place the eggplant in the water for several hours, until it begins to brown. Discard the eggplant (or dry it out and use it to cook with), and drink several ounces (up to 60) daily for several weeks.

Roasted Garlic (see page 151)

Several recent studies indicate that garlic is more effective than a placebo at decreasing blood pressure (Ried, et al, 2010; Ried, et al, 2008), although there are still some questions about these findings (Simons, et al, 2009). But garlic has all sorts of other benefits, and we are just crazy about it. It appears in many recipes throughout these pages.

Anti-Inflammatory Curcumin Scramble (see page 103)

Curcumin, the active ingredient in turmeric, has all sorts of healthful properties. There are some indications that its anti-inflammatory action may help reduce the risk of everything from acne to eczema to cancer. Some animal research suggests that it may also help fight hypertension and vascular tension (Morimoto, et al, 2008; Sompamit, et al, 2009). We've incorporated turmeric into many of our favorite dishes, from scrambled eggs (see above), to *Curry Soup* (see page 119) and *Curried Sweet Potato Fries* (see page 145), among others.

WARNING: Those taking the anticoagulant warfarin (Coumadin) should not take curcumin.

··· REFERENCES ···

Al-Solaiman, Y., Jesri, A., et al. "DASH lowers blood pressure in obese hypertensives beyond potassium, magnesium, and fibre." *Journal of Human Hypertension* 2009 Jul 23 [Epub ahead of print]

Appel, L. J., Moore, T. J., et al. "A clinical trial for the effects of dietary patterns on blood pressure. DASH Collaborative Research Group." *New England Journal of Medicine* 1997; 336(16): 1117-1124.

Blumenthal, J.A., Babyak, M.A., et al. "Effects of the DASH diet alone and in combination with exercise and weight loss on blood pressure and cardiovascular biomarkers in men and women with high blood pressure: the ENCORE study." *Archives of Internal Medicine* 2010 ; 170(2):126-35.

Buijsse, B., Weikert, C., et al. "Chocolate consumption in relation to blood pressure and risk of cardiovascular disease in German adults." *European Heart Journal* 2010; 31(13):1616-23. Epub 2010 Mar 30.

Desch, S., Kobler, D., et al. "Low vs. higher-dose dark chocolate and blood pressure in cardiovascular high-risk patients." *American Journal of Hypertension* 2010; 23(6):694-700. Epub 2010 Mar 4.

Grassi, D., Desideri, G., and Ferri, C. "Blood pressure and cardiovascular risk: What about cocoa and chocolate?" *Archives of Biochemistry and Biophysics* 2010 Jun 1. [Epub ahead of print]

He, Feng J., Markandu, Nirmala D., and MacGregor, Graham A. "Modest salt reduction lowers blood pressure in isolated systolic hypertension and combined hypertension." *Hypertension* 2005; 46:66.

Kapil, Vikas, Milsom, Alexandra B., et al. "Inorganic nitrate supplementation lowers blood pressure in humans: Role for nitrite-derived NO." *Hypertension* 2010; 56:274-281.

Kwon, Y. I., Apostolidis, E., and Shetty, K. "In vitro studies of eggplant (Solanum melongena) phenolics as inhibitors of key enzymes relevant for type 2 diabetes and hypertension." *Bioresource Technology* 2008; 99(8):2981-2988. [Epub 2007 Aug 13]

Morimoto, T., Sunagawa, Y., et al. "The dietary compound curcumin inhibits p300 histone acetyltransferase activity and prevents heart failure in rats." *The Journal of Clinical Investigation* 2008; 118(3):868-78.

Ried, K., Frank, O.R., and Stocks, N.P. "Aged garlic extract lowers blood pressure in patients with treated but uncontrolled hypertension: A randomised controlled trial." *Maturitas* 2010 Jun 29. [Epub ahead of print]

Ried, K., Sullivan, T., et al. "Does chocolate reduce blood pressure? A meta-analysis." BMC *Medicine* 2010 Jun 28; 8: 39.

Ried, K., Frank, O. R., et al. "Effect of garlic on blood pressure: a systematic review and meta-analysis." BMC *Cardiovascular Disorders* 2008; 8:13.

Sacks, F. M., Svetkey, L. P., et al. "Effects on blood pressure of reduced dietary sodium and the Dietary Approaches to Stop Hypertension (DASH) diet." *New England Journal of Medicine* 2001; 344:3-10.

Saftlas, A.F., Triche, E.W., et al. "Does chocolate intake during pregnancy reduce the risks of preeclampsia and gestational hypertension?" *Annals of Epidemiology* 2010; 20(8):584-91.

Simons, S., Wollersheim, H., and Thien, T. "A systematic review on the influence of trial quality on the effect of garlic on blood pressure." *Netherlands Journal of Medicine* 2009; 67(6): 212-9.

Sipahi, Ilke, Debanne, Sara M., et al. "Angiotensin-receptor blockade and risk of cancer: Meta-analysis of randomized controlled trials." *Lancet Oncology* 2010; 11(7):627-636.

Sompamit, K., Kukongviriyapan, U., et al. "Curcumin improves vascular function and alleviates oxidative stress in non-lethal lipopolysaccharide-induced endotoxaemia in mice." *European Journal of Pharmacology* 2009; 616(1-3):192-9. Epub 2009 Jun 17.

Webb, A., et al. "Acute blood pressure lowering, vasoprotective, and antiplatelet properties of dietary nitrate via bioconversion to nitrite." *Hypertension* 2008; 51:784.

··· DEALING WITH INDIGESTION ···

There is almost nothing as unpleasant as indigestion. It can come in many forms: constipation, diarrhea, gas, heartburn, and nausea can afflict anyone, and probably have at one time or another.

But sometimes, digestive distress can be far more serious: conditions like Crohn's disease, diverticulitis, gastrointestinal reflux disease (GERD), irritable bowel syndrome, and ulcerative colitis can severely affect one's quality of life. Diagnosis also often results in a prescription—sometimes forever, or at least that is the implication. And while certain drugs certainly can help make life more bearable for folks suffering from these disorders, some experts fear that medications may make things worse, not better. For instance, chronic use of proton pump inhibitors (PPIs) for GERD may lead to all sorts of dangerous side effects, from pneumonia (Laheij, et al, 2004) to an increased risk of fractures (Gray, et al, 2010) and a serious gastrointestinal infection, *Clostridium difficile* (Linsky, et al, 2010; Kim, et al, 2010). PPIs can also lead to rebound hyperacidity even in formerly healthy people when the medications are discontinued (Reimer, et al, 2009), which can make withdrawal unbearable.

No one should ever stop a course of treatment without the careful supervision of his physician, but it may be worthwhile to try altering a few things in your diet before reaching first for a pill bottle. Here are a few recipes, remedies, and suggestions for dietary changes that may help ameliorate the discomfort of digestive complaints.

··· CONSTIPATION ···

Power Pudding

Fluids and fiber are the two ingredients crucial for dealing with constipation. One recipe that incorporates both, and which many of our readers swear by, is Power Pudding.

> 1 cup coarse wheat bran
> 1 cup applesauce
> ¾ cup prune juice

Mix ingredients together and refrigerate. Take one to two tablespoons daily and wash it down with plenty of water.

Pumpkin Bran Muffins

Kit Gruelle gave us her recipe for delicious high-fiber muffins that combat constipation. Many readers of our column have benefited.
Preheat oven to 400 degrees.

> 1 cup whole wheat flour
> 1 ½ teaspoons baking powder
> ½ teaspoon baking soda
> 1 teaspoon cinnamon

> ½ teaspoon ground ginger
> 1 teaspoon nutmeg

Combine in a large mixing bowl and set aside.

> 2 cups bran cereal
> 1¼ cups reduced-fat milk
> ⅓ cup dark brown sugar
> 1 large egg
> ½ cup canned pumpkin
> ¾ cup raisins
> ½ cup diced dried apple

Combine in another bowl and stir well.

Let the bran mixture sit for approximately five minutes to allow the bran to soften. Stir in into the dry ingredients (in the large bowl). Don't overmix.

Drop the batter into muffin pans lightly oiled and lined with cupcake papers. Bake at 400 degrees for about 18 to 20 minutes, until a toothpick inserted in the center of a muffin comes out barely clean.

··· DIARRHEA ···

Coconut Macaroons

Listeners and readers have told us over the years that coconut was helpful for easing their diarrhea. And not just folks who've happened onto an unfortunate case of Montezuma's revenge while traveling overseas; even some longtime sufferers with Crohn's disease or ulcerative colitis have found surprising relief with this delicious fruit.

It can be consumed in the form of unsweetened, shredded coconut meat or as coconut milk. It can also be enjoyed in the form of cookies. We've heard from many people who swear by coconut macaroons—a couple per day seems to be a good initial dose for those with severe diarrhea. Just keep in mind that cookies tend to have a lot of calories, and while gaining weight may be something that a person suffering from chronic diarrhea may aspire to, lots of empty calories and refined carbohydrates aren't great for any of us. If you plan to ingest coconut regularly, we suggest mostly relying on milk or unsweetened meat. But every so often, nothing is tastier than a toothsome batch of cookies. Here is one recipe we received from Carolyn in Virginia:

> 2⅔ cups shredded coconut
> ⅔ cup sugar
> ¼ teaspoon salt
> 1 teaspoon almond extract
> 4 egg whites

Mix ingredients well, drop by teaspoonfuls on greased cookie sheet and bake for 20 minutes at 325 degrees (or until lightly brown). Remove immediately from cookie sheet when done.

Q *I have had colitis for almost three years. Last month a friend mentioned that she read an article in the newspaper about coconut macaroon cookies preventing diarrhea.*

I was ready to try anything, so I bought some cookies. The rest is history. I can now go anywhere without worrying about my uncontrollable problem! I consider it a miracle!

A We have heard from hundreds of readers about the benefits of dried coconut or macaroon cookies to combat chronic diarrhea. Whether the symptoms are from irritable bowel syndrome (IBS) or colitis, many people find this natural remedy helpful.

Dairy-Free Diet

Lactose intolerance is much more prevalent than many people realize. If you are troubled with indigestion, gas, bloating, or diarrhea, try giving up milk and other dairy products for several days and see what happens. If this makes a big difference for you, you may be lactose intolerant. (And if adding dairy back into your diet reintroduces the problem, then you can pretty much guarantee it.)

Even those who are not lactose intolerant may be interested to read the following recipe from Ayurvedic specialists the Mathises about drinking "super milk" in lieu of regular cold cow's milk:

"Super Milk"
Contributed by David Mathis, MD, FAAFP, ABHM, D.Ay.,
and Debbie Mathis, MA, D.Ay.

Soak 10 raw almonds overnight in water, then peel
and blend with:

1 cup organic unhomogenized cow's milk that has been
heated to boiling and cooled a bit
1 teaspoon ghee (clarified butter that can be found
at many health food stores)
1 teaspoon raw honey
Pinch of nutmeg
Pinch of saffron

Heat milk to the boiling point. Don't consume cold. Spice it with pinches of cinnamon, cardamom, ginger, and nutmeg. If you like, add a little honey (after heating, not before).

The Mathises explain the idea behind using "super milk" this way:

"There has long been debate about whether cow's milk is an appropriate food for humans. Convincing arguments exist on both sides of the question. If milk is a part of your diet, we would suggest some simple

Ayurvedic guidelines that can enhance milk's digestibility and help you avoid many of the problems associated with its consumption.

"With a few exceptions like the almonds in the recipe above and grains in general, milk should be consumed on its own. It should not be taken with other foods nor used as a beverage accompanying a meal.

"A nourishing and delicious drink containing the four substances (honey, almonds, ghee, and milk) recognized by Ayurvedic physicians as most supportive of the immune and reproductive systems, 'Super milk' can be taken in lieu of breakfast or a light evening meal.

"Use only organic, unhomogenized milk."

Yogurt and Probiotics
(See recipe for *Live & Active breakfast* on page 107)

Probiotics are healthy bacteria. Many people with chronic diarrhea have an unhealthy ratio of bad to good bacteria in their digestive systems, and eating yogurt with live and active cultures or taking probiotic supplements can help restore the balance. It may also help with other conditions that are often symptoms of a suppressed immune system, like eczema and acne. One study found that an anti-inflammatory medicine and a particular kind of probiotic (VSL#3) worked better for diverticulitis together than either did alone (Tursi, 2007).

··· GAS ···

Bitters

One remedy for gas is several generous sips of Angostura bitters. The following recipe may do double-duty on both digestive woes and muscle cramps, as the quinine in tonic water helps some people with the latter problem.

2 to 4 teaspoons Angostura bitters
8 ounces tonic water (or diet tonic water)

Mix ingredients vigorously, over ice if you like, and sip until feeling better. We've heard from some readers who prefer to mix the Angostura in club soda or 7-Up to mask the bitter taste, and other possibilities abound.

Angostura bitters do contain alcohol, so those avoiding alcohol should also avoid bitters.

Caraway Seed Tea

Caraway has long been used in other parts of the world to relieve flatulence. One easy and pleasant way to consume it is in the form of a tea.

1 teaspoon caraway seeds
8 ounces boiling water

Crush the seeds with a spoon to bruise them. Pour boiling water over them. Let steep for several minutes, strain out the seeds, and sweeten to taste as desired. Sip the tea two or three times daily.

Fennel Seed Tea

Like caraway seeds, fennel seeds have long been considered a digestive aid. In some Indian and South Asian restaurants, sugarcoated fennel seeds are offered at the end of a meal. They can also be sipped in the form of a tea that is quite similar to caraway seed tea.

½ teaspoon fennel seeds, smashed with the back of a spoon
8 ounces boiling water

Cover seeds with water and steep for five minutes. Strain out the seeds and sweeten to taste.

The Mathises have also shared with us a recipe for a delicious digestive tea that includes fennel and other seeds. The recipe for their digestive tea is below:

Digestive Tea
Contributed by David Mathis, MD, FAAFP, ABHM, D.Ay.,
and Debbie Mathis, MA, D.Ay.

½ teaspoon cumin seeds
½ teaspoon coriander seeds
½ teaspoon fennel seeds

Bring 8-12 ounces of water to a boil, add the seeds, and remove from heat. Allow to steep for five minutes. Strain and enjoy.

You can also mix a larger amount of seeds in equal parts and store in a glass jar. Use about 1 ½ teaspoons of the mix per cup.

The Mathises suggest: "If you experience gas, bloating or heaviness after eating, or if you simply want to improve your digestion of a meal, try this easy recipe. It's especially good whenever meat or cheese, both hard-to-digest foods, are on the menu."

Fennel Salad (see page 147)

Eating a bit of fresh fennel may have the same salubrious effect as drinking fennel seed tea, and it tastes delicious.

Yogurt and Probiotics (see DIARRHEA, above)

Broccoli and Garlic Stir Fry

One remedy for heartburn that may surprise you is broccoli. But in fact this delicious dark green vegetable contains a compound called sulforaphane that can kill tough intestinal bacteria like Helicobacter pylori (Lee, et al, 2008). This nasty bug can lead to stomach ulcers. That may be one reason some of our readers have reported relief from heartburn by eating broccoli. Broccoli has many other wonderful and healthful properties, too. For instance, some animal studies have shown that sulforaphane can reduce the number and size of colon polyps (Hu, et al, 2006). And it appears that cooking it with garlic may offer even more benefit. One recipe that accomplishes that tasty task is below.

> 2 cloves garlic, sliced thinly
> 2 tablespoons grapeseed or other high-heat cooking oil
> 1 large head broccoli, washed and cut into florets
> ¼ cup water
> 2 tablespoons soy sauce
> 1 tablespoon rice wine vinegar
> 1 teaspoon cornstarch
> 1 teaspoon crushed hot peppers (optional)

Heat the oil in a wok. While waiting for the oil to heat, whisk together the soy sauce, vinegar, cornstarch, and crushed peppers if desired, and stir until thickened.

Add the garlic to the oil. When sizzling, add the broccoli florets, and stir until coated in the garlic-infused oil. Add the water amd cover for a few minutes. Pour in the sauce, stir, turn the heat to low, and cook lidded until the broccoli are cooked through but still crunchy and bright green, about four or five minutes.

Ginger Pickle

*Contributed by David Mathis, MD, FAAFP, ABHM, D.Ay.,
and Debbie Mathis, MA, D.Ay.*

Another time-honored digestive aid is ginger, which has been used to treat bellyaches, nausea, and indigestion for hundreds if not thousands of years.

Peeled fresh ginger root
Fresh lime juice
Salt

Slice thin cross sections of ginger. Squeeze a little fresh lime juice over the slices, and lightly sprinkle them with salt.

To kick-start good digestion, eat about two slices per person, per meal, about 10-15 minutes before eating.

Here is the Mathises' explanation for the efficacy of this recipe:

"Everyone knows that good quality food is vital to wellbeing. Fresh food, in season, locally grown, and organic is definitely the way to go if possible. But the body's ability to digest that good food is the most overlooked part of a western diet. If the digestive fire is not strong, a toxic residue from even the best quality foods can create problems throughout the physiology. Protecting digestion is one of the most important aspects of achieving and maintaining health.

"Priming the pump with an easy-to-make little appetizer like ginger pickle will improve the digestive process and increase the absorption of nutrients."

Ginger Tea (see below, in NAUSEA)

Kitchari

Contributed by David Mathis, MD, FAAFP, ABHM, D.Ay.,
and Debbie Mathis, MA, D.Ay.

1 cup split yellow mung beans
1 cup white basmati rice
6 cups water
1 tablespoon fresh ginger root, peeled and minced
2-3 bay leaves
¼ teaspoon salt
3 tablespoons ghee (unsalted, clarified butter;
   available in many health food stores)
½ teaspoon turmeric (curcumin)
½ teaspoon cumin seeds
½ teaspoon fennel seeds
½ teaspoon mustard seeds
¼ to ½ cup chopped cilantro leaves,
   plus additional leaves for garnish
Unsweetened shredded coconut

Wash the beans in a strainer. (Soaking for an hour or more is good if you have the time, but skip this step if you don't.) Wash the rice in a strainer until the water runs clear.

Put both the beans and rice into a large pot or saucepan. Add the water, bay leaf, and minced ginger. Bring to a boil uncovered, skim off the foam, and turn the heat to low. Partially lid the pot, and stir occasionally to prevent sticking. Cook until tender and porridge-like, approximately 25-30 minutes. You may add more water for a thinner consistency if you prefer. When the kitchari is nearly done, add the salt.

Heat the ghee in a small sauté pan until liquefied. Add the turmeric, cumin, and fennel and mustard seeds to the ghee. When the mustard seeds begin to pop, pour the mixture into the kitchari, and stir in the cilantro leaves. Garnish as desired with coconut and more cilantro.

Here is the Mathises' explanation for the efficacy of this recipe:

"One of the most useful foods for health improvement is kitchari, a tasty combination of split yellow mung beans (also called split yellow mung dal) and white basmati rice, both widely available in health food stores, Asian markets and online. An excellent protein combination, it is both easy to digest and nourishing to all the tissues of the body. Kitchari gives strength and vitality, assisting in the recovery from illness or fatigue. It also improves digestive ability, making it an appropriate diet choice for cleansing programs. After a day of eating only kitchari (small amount for breakfast, largest amount mid-day and small amount in the evening), one's GI tract can more efficiently handle the harder-to-digest items of a 'normal' diet, thus reducing the toxic accumulations from poorly digested food."

Low-Carbohydrate Diet

We have heard stories from several of our listeners and readers who report that cutting refined sugars and simple carbohydrates from their diets helped them eliminate acid reflux. Some who had been on medication for years were even able to get off of it simply by switching to a low-carb diet. There are also some scientific data that support their experiences (Austin, et al, 2006).

We are certainly proponents of limiting intake of simple sugars and carbohydrates, as these foods can lead to all kinds of problems in addition to indigestion. Weight gain, for one, with its increased risk of diabetes and heart disease. But these foods also lead to inflammation, which may put people at a greater risk for everything from acne to eczema to cancer. So limiting your consumption of sugars and starches will benefit more than your gut.

Mustard and Vinegar Dressing (see page 9)

Q *I was prescribed Nexium for heartburn, but it began to lose its effectiveness and I worried about side effects. I found that yellow mustard worked faster and longer.*

A Nexium is a powerful and expensive way to treat routine heartburn. Many others have told us that yellow mustard can help ease heartburn. Other options include old-fashioned antacids such as baking soda or calcium carbonate, as well as home remedies such as a spoonful of vinegar or a few almonds after a meal.

Persimmon Punch

We first heard about using persimmons for heartburn several years ago, from a woman who was served persimmon punch during a meal at a Korean restaurant. She reported that it stopped her heartburn, and she started mixing up a batch at home. After several months of adding a few tablespoons to her morning and afternoon tea, she discovered that her cholesterol and blood sugar levels were also lower. Below is a recipe for persimmon punch:

> 2 quarts water
> ⅔ cup fresh ginger root, peeled and sliced
> 3 cinnamon sticks
> ½ cup honey
> 1 fresh, ripe persimmon, sliced thinly
>   (or substitute ½ cup dried sliced persimmons)

Add the ginger and cinnamon sticks to the water and bring to a boil. Turn the heat down and simmer it gently for 30 minutes. Strain the liquid and add the honey and persimmon. Refrigerate and enjoy cold. The tea will keep refrigerated for up to a week.

Yogurt and Probiotics (see DIARRHEA, above)

··· IRRITABLE BOWEL SYNDROME ···

Anti-Inflammatory Curcumin Scramble (see page 103)

Curcumin is the active ingredient in the spice turmeric, and it's what gives both curry and yellow mustard their bright color. It appears in many popular dishes around the world, and it has long

Q *For twenty-five years I have suffered with acid reflux and have taken strong acid-suppressing drugs, both prescription and over the counter.*

I have also suffered five fractures at different times and have osteoporosis of the spine. I had been an avid tennis player, swimmer and walker, in short, a physically active person.

I began taking probiotics several months ago and have had only one night of heartburn. I can sleep flat instead of sitting up. I can even bend over without the acid coming up. I have been cured!

A The FDA recently issued a caution that long-term use of acid-suppressing drugs may increase the risk of bone fractures. There is very little solid data on using probiotics for treating heartburn, but we are pleased you had such good results.

been thought to hold healthful properties. Recently, the medical literature has caught up, and over the past couple of decades, many studies confirming the health benefits of turmeric have been published. Most of these focus on its anti-inflammatory properties.

Researchers are only starting to understand the role inflammation plays in a variety of diseases, including everything from eczema to cancer to irritable bowel syndrome. We've heard anecdotal evidence from people who have found adding turmeric to their diets to be helpful for soothing symptoms of IBS. There is some research to support this claim (Bundy, et al, 2004), but the data are mixed; another study found that it worked no better than placebo (Brinkhaus, et al, 2005).

One thing that you should know if you're considering adding curcumin to your diet is that it may interact with the blood-thinner warfarin (Coumadin) to raise INR (a measure of blood coagulation).

WARNING: This can be very serious, so **anyone taking Coumadin should avoid turmeric.** Coumadin may also elevate liver enzymes in some people, which is a signal that the liver is having trouble processing it. If you decide to start ingesting curcumin regularly, you should be sure to consult your doctor and get your liver enzymes tested regularly. Finally, some people develop an allergic reaction to curcumin. If you get a rash or hives after eating it, you should stop.

But if these aren't concerns for you, there are lots of healthful and delicious ways to introduce more curcumin into your diet. One way is with the *Anti-Inflammatory Curcumin Scramble*, which we usually eat several times per week. You might also like to try our *Cancer-Fighting Cabbage Curry* (page 115), *Curry Soup* (page 119), or *Pork & Pineapple Curry with Coconut Chutney* (page 139).

Gluten-Free Diet

People with celiac disease are unable to digest gluten, which is a protein found in barley, wheat, and rye. More attention is being devoted to celiac disease in the media these days, but many sufferers still do not know that they have it, which often leads them—and even their doctors—to misdiagnose their symptoms. The gas, bloating, cramping, and diarrhea that is frequently identified as irritable bowel syndrome may in fact be disguising an inability to process gluten.

To find out if this is what has been troubling you, conduct a simple experiment: cut all gluten from your diet for at least a week or two. If you begin to feel better, you may have celiac disease, particularly if your symptoms return upon reintroduction of foods containing gluten.

Celiac disease is quite serious, so if you suspect that you may have it, you should get a formal diagnosis and alter your diet accordingly. Do not eliminate gluten before your test; the results may not be accurate if you do. There are now many cookbooks and prepared foods specifically for people who must avoid gluten.

··· NAUSEA ···

Ginger Tea

Ginger is a time-honored remedy for nausea, and there is some evidence that it may be useful for those experiencing everything from motion sickness (Lien, et al, 2003) to morning sickness (Borrelli, et al, 2005; Ozgoli, et al, 2009) to chemotherapy-induced nausea (Levine, et al, 2008), although in the last instance, the ginger was taken in combination with a high-protein meal, which may have been at least as responsible for the reduction in symptoms.

Ginger can be taken in many forms: in capsules, in ginger ale or beer, in ginger snaps, as candy, like crystallized ginger or ginger chews, or in a tasty tea. A recipe for ginger tea follows:

1 piece of fresh ginger root that's about
as big as your thumb, peeled
8 ounces boiling water

Grate the ginger into a mug. Pour the boiling water over it. Allow the mixture to steep for roughly five minutes, strain, and sweeten to taste.

··· REFERENCES ···

Austin, Gregory L., Thiny, Michelle T., et al. "A very low-carbohydrate diet improves gastroesophageal reflux and its symptoms." *Digestive Diseases and Sciences* 2006; 51(8):1307-1312.

Borrelli, F., Capasso, R., et al. "Effectiveness and safety of ginger in the treatment of pregnancy-induced nausea and vomiting." *Obstetrics & Gynecology* 2005; 105(4):849-856.

Brinkhaus, B., Hentschel, C., et al. "Herbal medicine with curcuma and fumitory in the treatment of irritable bowel syndrome: A randomized, placebo-controlled, double-blind clinical trial." *Scandinavian Journal of Gastroenterology* 2005; 40(8):936-943.

Bundy, R., Walker, A. F., et al. "Turmeric extract may improve irritable bowel syndrome symptomology in otherwise healthy adults: A pilot study." *Journal of Alternative and Complementary Medicine* 2004; 10(6):1015-1018.

Gray, S.L., LaCroix, A.Z., et al. "Proton pump inhibitor use, hip fracture, and change in bone mineral density in postmenopausal women: results from the Women's Health Initiative." *Archives of Internal Medicine.* 2010; 170(9):765-771.

Hu, R., et al. "Cancer chemoprevention of intestinal polyposis in Apc-Min/+ mice by sulforaphane, a natural product derived from cruciferous vegetables." *Carcinogenesis* 2006; 27(10):2038-2046.

Katz, M.H. "Failing the acid test: benefits of proton pump inhibitors may not justify the risks for many users." *Archives of Internal Medicine.* 2010; 170(9):747-748.

Kim, J.W., Lee, K.L., et al. "Proton pump inhibitors as a risk factor for recurrence of *Clostridium-difficile*-associated diarrhea." *World Journal of Gastroenterology.* 2010; 16(28):3573-3577.

Laheij, R.J., Sturkenboom, M.C., et al. "Risk of community-acquired pneumonia and use of gastric acid-suppressive drugs." *Journal of the American Medical Association.* 2004; 292(16):1955-1960.

Lee, S. Y., Shin, Y. W., and Hahm K. B. "Phytoceuticals: Mighty but ignored weapons against *Helicobacter pylori* infection." *Journal of Digestive Diseases* 2008; 9(3):129-139.

Levine, M.E., Gillis, M.G., et al. "Protein and ginger for the treatment of chemotherapy-induced delayed nausea." *Journal of Alternative & Complementary Medicine* 2008; 14(5):545-551.

Lien, H. C., Sun, W. M., et al. "Effects of ginger on motion sickness and gastric slow-wave dysrhythmias induced by circular vection." *American Journal of Physiology—Gastrointestinal and Liver Physiology* 2003; 284(3):G481-G489.

Linsky, A., Gupta, K., et al. "Proton pump inhibitors and risk for recurrent *Clostridium difficile* infection." *Archives of Internal Medicine* 2010; 170(9):772-778.

Ozgoli, G., Goli, M., and Simbar, M. "Effects of ginger capsules on pregnancy, nausea, and vomiting." *Journal of Alternative & Complementary Medicine* 2009; 15(3):243-246.

Reimer, C., Søndergaard, B., et al. "Proton-pump inhibitor therapy induces acid-related symptoms in healthy volunteers after withdrawal of therapy." *Gastroenterology.* 2009; 137(1): 80-7, 87.e1. Epub 2009 Apr 10.

Tursi, A., Brandimarte, G., et al. "Balsalazide and/or high-potency probiotic mixture (VSL#3) in maintaining remission after attack of acute, uncomplicated diverticulitis of the colon." *International Journal of Colorectal Disease* 2007; 22(9):1103-1108.

··· COMBATING JOINT PAIN
AND ARTHRITIS ···

Joint pain tends to trouble a lot of us as we get older. Arthritis, gout, and other painful conditions can make standing, sitting, and just about everything else excruciating.

There are a lot of unknowns about why joints become inflamed. We don't know why some people develop osteoarthritis in their sixties, fifties, or even their forties while other people dance along into their nineties without ever suffering soreness in their joints. We don't know why runners and other athletes who put lots of stress and strain on their bones don't seem to develop more arthritis than other folks. Researchers also don't know why arthritis sometimes seems to crop up as a direct reaction to something—a case of salmonella poisoning, for instance. And they also know very little about what causes rheumatoid arthritis, an extremely painful chronic condition.

Many people lean heavily on non-steroidal anti-inflammatories (NSAIDS) like ibuprofen and naproxen to get through the day. These over-the-counter pharmaceuticals do work quite well to temporarily alleviate pain and inflammation, but it's easy to forget that they're powerful drugs—not meant to be taken daily nor at the dosages that many people ingest. According to surveys by Roper and the National Consumers League, more than 20 million Americans take NSAIDs every day (Wilcox, et al, 2005). Of those, about a quarter take more than the recommended dose, and about half don't know that NSAIDs can potentially be harmful.

But they can be. Among other things, they can increase a person's risk for a heart attack or stroke, raise blood pressure, and irritate the GI tract, which can lead to bleeding ulcers. As a result, people who are aware of the risks have begun searching elsewhere for pain relief, and many have sent us their recipes and remedies for alternative therapies.

Anti-Inflammatory Curcumin Scramble (see page 103)

It has been well established in the scientific literature that curcumin, the active ingredient in turmeric, has amazing anti-inflammatory activities. Type "curcumin" and "anti-inflammatory" into the database PubMed and more than 650 results will pop up. One recent animal study suggested that curcumin might help to reduce inflammation in the joints of arthritic mice (Moon, et al, 2010).

A number of the recipes in this book contain curcumin. See, for instance: *Curry Soup* (page 119), *Curried Sweet Potato Fries* (page 145), and *Cancer-Fighting Cabbage Curry* (page 115).

WARNING: Curcumin is also available in supplement form. **Those taking the blood-thinner warfarin (Coumadin) should avoid curcumin.**

Recipe 1: Curcumin Milk

Put a mug's worth of milk on the stove and bring to boil. While it's heating, put a small amount of room temperature milk in your mug and add 1 teaspoon of turmeric, 1 teaspoon of honey (or less—to taste), and a sprinkle of ground black pepper. Mix well. When the milk on the stove has boiled, add it to the mixture, stir again, and enjoy. If you are diabetic, skip the honey and add a sprinkle of cinnamon to the milk.

The curcumin in turmeric is insoluble in water but totally soluble in dairy fats. The idea behind the pepper is that it contains piperine, which will boost absorption of the curcumin considerably.

Recipe 2

If you cannot drink milk, try sprinkling 1 teaspoon of turmeric on your toast, spread on plenty of very ripe avocado (the oil in the avocado will make the curcumin soluble), and sprinkle with salt and pepper to taste.

Certo & Grape Juice

Certo is a fruit pectin that comes in a gelatin powder. Although we don't really understand how it works, we have now heard from literally dozens if not hundreds of people who say that mixing Certo with purple Concord grape juice works to help relieve their joint pain. There are a few different recipes, but a standard one we've heard is below.

"I was misdiagnosed with polymyalgia rheumatica and given massive doses of prednisone for years. It wasn't until I found a pain specialist who hates prednisone that I finally weaned myself off of it. But I still had lots of muscle and joint pain. Then I heard about turmeric and decided to try it.

After doing lots of research, I found a recipe that works very well to relieve my pain. If you're able to free yourself from a drug mentality and don't expect it to work overnight, you will be very surprised by the results within a few weeks.

I have been taking curcumin regularly for one month, and have increased mobility and a lot less pain. I'm now on no medication at all."

1 tablespoon Certo
8 ounces grape juice

Thoroughly mix the Certo powder into the grape juice and consume daily.

"I was experiencing such terrible joint pain that I had trouble bending my leg enough to put on my sock. I climbed stairs like a small child, mounting one step with my right foot, bringing my left to the same step, then repeating with my right foot one more step, and

In desperation, I decided to try grape juice with Certo. I planned to try it for a month. Within just three days, I was putting on my socks with no difficulty. Yesterday, I found myself climbing stairs normally.

I understand that nobody knows how this works, and I am a skeptic, but it does work. Not incidentally, I am 89 years old."

Alternative: for those who don't like grape juice, pomegranate juice seems to work just as well, if not better, as a substitute.

Cherry Spritzer

There has been some research conducted on animals indicating that anthocyanins in cherries, the compounds that make them red, have anti-inflammatory properties (He et al, 2006), and a study on humans from 1950 suggested that cherries could be useful for relieving pain from gout and arthritis. There was also a small study published in the *Journal of Nutrition* (Jacob, et al, 2003) that seemed to show sweet cherries could bring down the uric acid levels that lead to gout. But while the scientific data are somewhat lacking, we have gathered lots of anecdotal evidence from folks who claim that cherries have done wonders to relieve their joint pain. Cherries can be purchased in the form of concentrated cherry capsules, as supplement bars, as both fresh and concentrated juice, and of course as fruit. Cherry juice concentrate is generally the least expensive of all of these options (though it too can be a bit pricey). One tasty recipe for a refreshing cherry juice spritzer is below.

2 tablespoons tart cherry juice concentrate
8 ounces sparkling water
Wedge of lime
Non-calorie sweetener to taste (optional)

Mix together the cherry juice concentrate, sparkling water, and sweetener, if desired, and add a squirt of fresh lime juice. Enjoy two glasses per day, or a bit more or less as needed for pain relief.

Fish & Fish Oil

It seems we can add pain relief to the many benefits of taking fish oil. There have been several studies indicating that it is good for the joints of rheumatoid arthritis (RA) sufferers. It also seems that patients who take fish oil take fewer NSAIDs. This is particularly good news for those with RA, as RA carries an increased risk of cardiovascular death, and NSAIDs only increase that risk (see, i.e., James, et al, 2010).

Some recipes in this book that contain fish or fish oil are: *Joe's Brain-Boosting Smoothie* (see page 107), *Spicy Fresh Tuna Salad* (see page 143), *Pescado al Cilantro* (see page 137), *Favorite Fish Platter* (see page 106), *Fish Tacos with Radish and Lime* (see page 120), *Salmon with Fava Bean and Spring Pea Mash* (see page 141), and *Horseradish Crusted Salmon with Cranberry Catsup* (see page 127).

Gin-Soaked Raisins

Another mysterious remedy that many of our readers and listeners swear by for joint pain relief is golden raisins soaked in gin.

8 ounces golden raisins
6 to 8 ounces gin

In a shallow pan, barely cover golden raisins with gin. Let them sit until the gin has completely evaporated. Eat 9 raisins per day.

It may take several weeks to experience results.

Virgin Raisins

For those who are avoiding alcohol, we received this recipe for non-alcoholic raisins on our website:

> 8 ounces golden raisins
> ½ cup apple cider vinegar
> ¼ cup honey

Stir the vinegar and honey until thoroughly mixed. Then follow the instructions for gin raisins above, substituting the vinegar-honey mixture for the gin.

Q *I suffered from tendinitis in my elbows and forearms for years. My doctor had tried several anti-inflammatory drugs and I had also followed his instructions for alternating hot and cold compresses. Nothing worked, and we were talking about surgery.*

A relative told me about golden raisins soaked in gin for tendinitis. I was ready to try almost anything, so I followed his advice.

Within a few weeks, I no longer had pain. I continued taking a spoonful a day for a couple of years and then stopped because I started a low-carb diet. Soon the tendinitis returned. When I resumed the raisins daily, the pain went away and hasn't returned.

A We can't explain how gin-soaked raisins relieve inflammation, but many readers have found them helpful for arthritis.

Gluten-Free Diet

Those with celiac disease are unable to digest gluten, a protein found in wheat, barley, and rye. One symptom of celiac disease can be joint pain. Try cutting gluten from your diet for several weeks to see if your pain subsides. If it does (and especially if it returns when you add gluten back into your diet), there is a good chance that you might have celiac disease, and you should visit your doctor for a proper diagnosis.

Pineapple-Cherry Cocktail

Bromelain is an enzyme found in pineapples that appears to have anti-inflammatory activity. Unfortunately, studies on its use for arthritis pain have been mixed. One showed that a product containing bromelain (Phlogenzym) helped ease pain from hip arthritis (Klein, et al, 2006), but another showed that it worked no better than placebo for knee arthritis (Brien, et al, 2006). We doubt that just eating pineapple will help ease pain, but perhaps this pineapple-cherry juice cocktail in combination with a bromelain-containing supplement might help for some people.

> 2 tablespoons cherry juice concentrate
> 8 ounces pineapple juice

Mix ingredients together and enjoy one to two glasses daily. (Keep in mind that fruit juice contains a lot of calories, so you may wish to adjust your diet accordingly.)

Vinegar & Honey

One of our readers told us he got the following recipe from a former owner of the Dallas Cowboys. He's in his eighties, and he swears by this combination to keep joint pain at bay.

½ teaspoon apple cider vinegar
½ teaspoon honey
1 teaspoon orange-flavored powdered gelatin
6 ounces water

Mix ingredients together thoroughly and drink at least one glass per day. If you're having trouble getting the ingredients to combine nicely, you can also mix the vinegar and honey together separately, and then add one teaspoon of the vinegar-honey mixture to the water and gelatin powder.

Virgin Mary

Some people swear by cayenne powder as an arthritis remedy. One way to make swallowing it more palatable may be to mix it in tomato juice or Bloody Mary Mix.

1 teaspoon cayenne pepper powder
6 ounces tomato juice or Bloody Mary Mix

Stir together and drink one small glass daily.

Alternative: if you don't like tomato juice, another rather odd combination we've heard is to mix the cayenne powder into orange juice: ¼ teaspoon in about 12 ounces of OJ.

··· REFERENCES ···

Brien, S., Lewith, G., et al. "Bromelain as an adjunctive treatment for moderate-to-severe osteoarthritis of the knee: a randomized placebo-controlled pilot study." *Quarterly Journal of Medicine* 2006; 99(12):841-850.

He, Y-H., et al. "Anti-inflammatory and anti-oxidative effects of cherries on Freund's adjuvant-induced arthritis in rats." *Scandinavian Journal of Rheumatology* 2006; 35(5):356–358.

Jacob, R.A., Spinozzi, G.M., et al. "Consumption of cherries lowers plasma urate in healthy women." *Journal of Nutrition* 2003; 133(6):1826-1829.

James, M., Proudman, S., and Cleland, L. "Fish oil and rheumatoid arthritis: Past, present and future." *Proceedings of the Nutrition Society* 2010; 69(3):316-323. Epub 2010 May 28.

Klein, G., Kullich, W., et al. "Efficacy and tolerance of an oral enzyme combination in painful osteoarthritis of the hip. A double-blind, randomised study comparing oral enzymes with non-steroidal anti-inflammatory drugs." *Clinical and Experimental Rheumatology* 2006; 24(1): 25-30.

Moon, D.O., Kim, M.O., et al. "Curcumin attenuates inflammatory response in IL-1beta-induced human synovial fibroblasts and collagen-induced arthritis in mouse model." *International Immunopharmacology* 2010; 10(5):605-610. Epub 2010 Feb 23.

Wilcox, C.M., Cryer, B., and Triadafilopoulos, G. "Patterns of use and public perception of over-the-counter pain relievers: Focus on non-steroidal antiinflammatory drugs." *Journal of Rheumatology* 2005; 32(11):2218-2224.

··· BOOSTING MEMORY ···

Losing our mental edge is something we all fear. Forgetfulness is a natural consequence of getting older, but we'd all like to sustain our cognitive firepower for as long as possible, and some exciting research on certain antioxidant-rich foods suggests that what we include in our diets may help in that endeavor.

James Joseph, PhD, a neuroscientist at Tufts University's Jean Mayer USDA Human Nutrition Research Center on Aging, did some fascinating animal and human studies regarding which foods enhance memory. Berries, and blueberries in particular, were at the center of much of his research, as in the case of one recent small study conducted by Dr. Joseph and several colleagues. It looked at the effects of daily blueberry juice consumption for nine older adults who showed some signs of memory problems. After three months, the people in the study did better on memory tests than a group drinking a placebo juice (Krikorian, et al, April 2010). Other benefits seemed to be some reversal of depression symptoms and better blood glucose levels.

In another study, Dr. Joseph found that along with berries, Concord grape juice and walnuts also appear to boost cognitive function in the aging brain (Joseph, et al, 2009). Indeed, Concord grape juice seems like it might help even those older adults who are already starting to experience problems with memory (Krikorian, et al, March 2010). Dr. Joseph and his colleague have published a raft of such studies on the positive cognitive effects of various berries and walnuts in animals and humans (see, i.e.: Shukitt-Hale, et al, 2009; Shukitt-Hale, et al, 2008; Willis, et al, January 2009; Willis, et al, April 2009). The berries don't need to be fresh to work—frozen berries and berry juice will work just as well. Two of our favorite berry recipes follow.

Joe's Brain-Boosting Smoothie (see page 107)

We love this smoothie and incorporate it into our breakfast rotation at least once or twice each week.

Q *I've heard that blueberries have a beneficial effect on the brain. Can you tell me more about this? Is the research recent and credible?*

A James Joseph, PhD, at Tufts University was a leading neuroscientist and expert on the effects of berries on brain function. He did a number of studies in both aging rodents and humans demonstrating cognitive benefits from blueberries (Krikorian, et al, April, 2010). Dr. Joseph recommended frozen berries as an economical way to get the antioxidant potential of this fruit.

Blueberry Cheesecake (see page 156)

Contributed by Steven Zeisel, MD, PhD
and Susan Zeisel, Ed.D.

While we don't recommend eating cheesecake daily as a way to boost brain power, this is a delicious dessert. It is also rich in choline, essential for brain health.

Certo & Grape Juice (see page 61)

For those who also suffer from joint pain, this recipe may kill two birds with one stone!

Favorite Fish Platter (see page 106)

Another food that may serve the brain is fish. One recent study that looked at nearly 15,000 older people in seven different countries (China, Cuba, the Dominican Republic, India, Mexico, Peru, and Venezuela) found that those who ate more fish were less likely to suffer from dementia (Albanese, et al, 2009).

We are very fond of fish and try to eat it several times per week. You'll find several recipes throughout these pages that incorporate a variety of fish: *Spicy Fresh Tuna Salad* (see page 143), *Pescado al Cilantro* (see page 137), *Fish Tacos with Radish and Lime* (see page 120), *Salmon with Fava Bean and Spring Pea Mash* (see page 141), and *Horseradish Crusted Salmon with Cranberry Catsup* (see page 127).

ONE CAUTION: the FDA has warned that large fish like shark, swordfish, king mackerel, and tilefish may contain unsafe levels of mercury. People and especially pregnant women should also limit their intake of tuna for the same reason. Fish oil capsules, however, should not contain mercury. (You can visit consumerlab.com for more information on tests of fish oil capsules. And for information on which fish are safest to consume, both for you and for the environment, Sea Food Watch from the Monterey Aquarium is a great resource. Visit: www.seafoodwatch.org.)

Lentil Nut Loaf with
Red Pepper Sauce (see page 135)

Contributed by Gail Pettiford Willett
and Walter Willett, MD, DrPH

We love this wonderful recipe, not least because it contains lots of walnuts, which have been shown to be excellent brain food.

Gluten-Free Diet

Celiac disease is an inability to digest gluten, a protein found in barley, rye, and wheat. One possible symptom is cognitive fuzziness. If you suspect you may have celiac disease, you should visit a doctor for testing and diagnosis. Celiac is quite serious, and for those suffering from it, cutting gluten from one's diet can make a big difference in all kinds of ways.

Mediterranean Diet

Another dietary approach that may protect against Alzheimer's disease is the Mediterranean diet. Several studies have shown that a Mediterranean-style diet leads to a statistically significant decrease in Alzheimer's diagnosis (Féart, et al, 2009; Scarmeas, et al, 2009; Sofi, et al, 2010). The Mediterranean diet incorporates lots of fresh vegetables and fruits, beans and legumes, lean sources of protein like fish, and it utilizes olive oil (vs. butter, for example) as its main source of dietary fat. For more information on the Mediterranean Diet, visit the Mayo Clinic's website at: http://www.mayoclinic.com/health/mediterranean-diet/CL00011. We have also included a section on this and other diets in our books *Favorite Foods from the People's Pharmacy* (2009) and *The People's Pharmacy Quick and Handy Home Remedies*, which will be published by National Geographic in 2011.

··· REFERENCES ···

Albanese, E., Dangour, A.D,. et al. "Dietary fish and meat intake and dementia in Latin America, China, and India: a 10/66 Dementia Research Group population-based study." *American Journal of Clinical Nutrition* 2009; 90: 392-400.

Féart, C., Samieri, C., et al. "Adherence to a Mediterranean diet, cognitive decline, and risk of dementia." *JAMA* 2009; 302: 638-648.

Joseph, J.A., Shukitt-Hale, B., and Willis, L.M. "Grape juice, berries, and walnuts affect brain aging and behavior." *Journal of Nutrition* 2009; 139(9): 1813S-1817S. Epub 2009 Jul 29.

Krikorian, R., Nash, T.A., et al. "Concord grape juice supplementation improves memory function in older adults with mild cognitive impairment." *British Journal of Nutrition* 2010 Mar; 103(5): 730-4. Epub 2009 Dec 23.

Krikorian, R., Shidler, M.D., et al. "Blueberry supplementation improves memory in older adults." *Journal of Agricultural and Food Chemistry* 2010 Apr 14; 58(7): 3996-4000.

Lau, F. C., Shukitt-Hale, B., and Joseph, J. A. "The beneficial effects of fruit polyphenols on brain aging." *Neurobiology of Aging* 2005; 26 Supp 1:128-132.

Scarmeas, N., Luchsinger, J.A., et al. "Physical activity, diet, and risk of Alzheimer disease." *JAMA* 2009; 302(6):627-637.

Shukitt-Hale, B., Lau, F.C., and Joseph, J.A. "Berry fruit supplementation and the aging brain." *Journal of Agricultural and Food Chemistry* 2008; 56(3):636-641. Epub 2008 Jan 23.

Shukitt-Hale, B., Cheng, V., Joseph, J.A. "Effects of blackberries on motor and cognitive function in aged rats." *Nutritional Neuroscience* 2009; 12(3):135-140.

Sofi, F., Macchi, C., et al. "Effectiveness of the Mediterranean diet: Can it help delay or prevent Alzheimer's disease?" *Journal of Alzheimer's Disease* 2010; 20(3):795-801.

Suh, S. J., Koo, B. S., et al. "Pharmacological characterization of orally active cholinesterase inhibitory activity of *Prunus persica* L. Batsch in rats." *Journal of Molecular Neuroscience* 2006; 29(2):101-107.

Willis, L.M., Shukitt-Hale, B., and Joseph, J.A. "Recent advances in berry supplementation and age-related cognitive decline." *Current Opinion in Clinical Nutrition & Metabolic Care* 2009 Jan; 12(1):91-94.

Willis, L.M., Shukitt-Hale, B., et al. "Dose-dependent effects of walnuts on motor and cognitive function in aged rats." *British Journal of Nutrition* 2009 Apr; 101(8):1140-1144.

···TACKLING SKIN CONDITIONS···

While skin conditions are rarely very dangerous, they can certainly affect one's quality of life and self-esteem. Eczema can itch like the dickens, as can psoriasis, and both can cause unsightly red patches on the skin that many find embarrassing. Both eczema and psoriasis are caused by an immune system gone slightly haywire. And some researchers think the same is true of acne.

It certainly seems likely that all three of these unpleasant conditions are affected in one way or another by diet. A recent crop of studies has drawn a link between acne and a diet laden with dairy and high-glycemic-index foods (Ferdowsian and Levin, 2010; Melnik and Schmitz, 2009). We've also heard anecdotal evidence from people who have seen an improvement of their eczema symptoms by avoiding dairy, gluten, soy, and foods with a high glycemic index.

We think it makes good sense for those hoping to get their skin under control to try steering clear of simple carbs and other foods that cause inflammation. It may help to add certain foods, beverages, and seasonings to your diet, too. Below are some recipes for fighting inflammation that may help with a variety of ailments that affect the skin.

Caraway Seed Tea for Rosacea

We've heard from some of our readers with rosacea that caraway seed tea has helped take away the redness in their skin. Rosacea is unrelated to acne, eczema, or psoriasis, but it, too, is caused by inflammation.

> 1 teaspoon caraway seeds, crushed with a spoon
> 8 ounces boiling water
> Sweetener to taste (optional)

Pour boiling water over the seeds. Let steep for up to 10 minutes. Strain out the seeds, and add sweetener to taste if desired. People sip this tea two or three times daily for relief of rosacea symptoms.

Fish & Fish Oil for Eczema

There has been a strong case made for the anti-inflammatory effects of fish and fish oil. These effects seem to extend to the treatment of eczema. Recently, some interesting research seems to indicate that children exposed to fish and fish oil in utero and infancy are less likely than other children to develop eczema later in childhood (Alm, et al, 2009; Calder, et al, 2010; Kremmyda, et al, 2010; Oien, et al, 2010). We've also heard from many adult eczema sufferers who find that their symptoms can be tamed by consumption of more fish and fish oil.

Some recipes in this book that contain fish or fish oil are: *Joe's Brain-Boosting Smoothie* (see page 107), *Spicy Fresh Tuna Salad* (see page 143), *Pescado al Cilantro* (see page 137), *Favorite Fish Platter* (see page 106), *Fish Tacos with Radish and Lime* (see page 120), *Salmon with Fava Bean and Spring Pea Mash* (see page 141), and

Horseradish Crusted Salmon with Cranberry Catsup (see page 127).

The FDA has warned people that large fish like shark, swordfish, king mackerel, and tilefish may contain unsafe levels of mercury. Pregnant women in particular should heed these warnings, and should limit their intake of tuna for the same reason. And anyone considering giving fish to a very young child should absolutely consult her pediatrician first.

Live & Active for Eczema (see page 107)

When contending with eczema symptoms, flaxseed and the probiotics in yogurt may also be helpful. Like fish and fish oil, flaxseed contains omega-3 fatty acids, shown to have anti-inflammatory properties. And some studies have shown probiotics to be useful for dealing with eczema in very young children (Grüber et al, 2007; Niers, 2009; Passeron et al, 2006). Again, though, we recommend talking to your pediatrician before introducing new things into your infant's diet.

But for adults, one tasty way to combine both probiotic-containing yogurt and flaxseed is in a delicious and healthy breakfast, like our *Live & Active*.

Curry Soup for Psoriasis (see page 119)

Psoriasis is a chronic condition for which there is no real cure. But it can certainly vary a great deal in severity. Curcumin, the active ingredient in the yellow spice turmeric, has powerful anti-inflammatory activity that has been shown to help block the enzyme PhK that is associated with the overactive cell growth responsible for psoriasis (Heng, et al, 2000). And while consuming more curcumin won't necessarily help everyone who suffers from psoriasis, it is safe for nearly everyone to try.

WARNING: The exception is those who take the anticoagulant warfarin (Coumadin), who should avoid curcumin.

We've included a number of recipes containing turmeric throughout these pages. See, for instance: *Anti-Inflammatory Curcumin Scramble* (page 103), *Pork & Pineapple Curry* (see page 139), *Curried Sweet Potato Fries* (page 145), and *Cancer-Fighting Cabbage*

Q *For a year and a half, my dermatologist has treated me for psoriasis. First I took cyclosporine and then CellCept.*

Like another reader stated, I too developed every side effect listed in the warnings I got with the medication: hair loss, blisters, dry skin and scalp, and blurred vision. Worst of all, I got no permanent relief from psoriasis!

I then tried a turmeric capsule twice a day (one in the a.m. and one at bed time), following your reader's example. Within two weeks, all my psoriasis patches disappeared and my hair loss has all but stopped! I don't even have the 24-hour heartburn I had on both cyclosporine and CellCept.

I cannot believe that with all the possible side effects of the two pricey prescriptions I was taking, such as lymphoma, liver failure and even death, my dermatologist did not suggest turmeric. Maybe it is because this spice found in curry powder can be purchased without a prescription at any health food store. I have not experienced any adverse side effects with the turmeric capsules.

A Many people with psoriasis find that turmeric or its active component curcumin can be helpful. Not everyone gets benefit, however, and some people develop a severe rash. No one taking the anticoagulant Coumadin (warfarin) should take turmeric medicinally. We have received several reports of excessive bleeding or high INR values from people combining these therapies. INR is a measure of bleeding susceptibility.

Curry (page 115). Turmeric is the ingredient in mustard that makes it yellow, so you could try consuming more mustard, as well, like our *Mustard and Vinegar Dressing* (see page 9). Curcumin can also be consumed in supplement form. And some folks with psoriasis have experimented with putting a turmeric poultice right on their skin—but be careful! It will dye everything it touches a very bright yellow, including skin.

··· REFERENCES ···

Alm, B., Aberg, N., et al. "Early introduction of fish decreases the risk of eczema in infants." *Archives of Disease in Childhood* 2009; 94(1):11-15. Epub 2008 Sep 25.

Calder, P.C., Kremmyda, L.S., et al. "Is there a role for fatty acids in early life programming of the immune system?" *Proceedings of the Nutrition Society* 2010; 69(3):373-380. [Epub 2010 May 13.]

Ferdowsian, H.R. and Levin, S. "Does diet really affect acne?" *Skin Therapy Letter* 2010; 15(3):1-2, 5.

Grüber, C., Wendt, M., et al. "Randomized, placebo-controlled trial of Lactobacillus rhamnosus GG as treatment of atopic dermatitis in infancy." *Allergy* 2007; 62(11):1270-1276.

Heng, M. C., Song, M. K., et al. "Drug-induced suppression of phosphorylase kinase activity correlates with resolution of psoriasis as assessed by clinical, histological and immunohistochemical parameters." *British Journal of Dermatology* 2000; 143(5):937-949.

Kremmyda, L.S., Vlachava, M., et al. "Atopy risk in infants and children in relation to early exposure to fish, oily fish, or long-chain omega-3 fatty acids: a systematic review." *Clinical Reviews in Allergy and Immunology* 2009 Dec 9. [Epub ahead of print]

Melnik, B. C., and Schmitz, G. "Role of insulin, insulin-like growth factor-1, hyperglycaemic food and milk consumption in the pathogenesis of acne vulgaris." *Experimental Dermatology* 2009; 18(10):833-841. [Epub ahead of print Aug. 25, 2009]

Niers, L., Martín, R., et al. "The effects of selected probiotic strains on the development of eczema (the PandA study)." *Allergy* 2009; 64(9):1349-1358. [Epub ahead of print].

Oien, T., Storrø, O., and Johnsen, R. "Do early intake of fish and fish oil protect against eczema and doctor-diagnosed asthma at 2 years of age? A cohort study." *Journal of Epidemiology and Community Health* 2010 Feb; 64(2):124-129. [Epub 2009 Aug 6.]

Passeron, T., Lacour, J. P., et al. "Prebiotics and synbiotics: Two promising approaches for the treatment of atopic dermatitis in children above 2 years." *Allergy* 2006; 61(4):431-437.

··· WEIGHT LOSS ···

The calculus for weight loss is deceptively simple: eat less; exercise more. Unfortunately, it's not that easy for most of us. If it were, no one would be overweight, which is obviously far from the case. And it's true that obesity increases the risk of many chronic conditions, from diabetes, high blood pressure and heart disease to certain types of cancer. For someone who is simply moderately overweight, losing as little as ten pounds can make a big difference in overall health.

But it's also true that being healthy is not just a matter of losing weight. It's certainly possible to be thin and unhealthy, and there are also plenty of people in excellent shape who are perhaps a bit heavier than their doctors would like them to be. More experts are starting to concede that it's better to be a bit heavy and exercising regularly than to be thin and unable to walk up a flight of stairs without wheezing (Neighmond, 2010). Indeed, there's more research amassing that just exercise alone is probably not enough to help people lose weight (Melanson, et al, 2009), although it appears that it will help a person keep pounds off if they do manage to lose (MacLean, et al, 2009). And the benefits of exercise are so significant and so diverse that weight loss should not be the main goal of incorporating more of it into our lifestyles (King, et al, 2009).

As you've probably guessed, though, if the key to losing weight isn't exercise per se, then it must be diet. And indeed it is. Changing the types of foods we eat, as well as the quantities in which we consume them (Clark, et al, 2010) is really what's required when it comes to losing weight. As a result, we unfortunately can't offer up a simple set of recipes or remedies that will make it easier. But one of the main reasons that we conceived of this book in the first place was to offer our thoughts on what a healthy, well-rounded diet would look like in a very literal and direct way. We can't promise that if you follow our meal plans for two weeks, you will lose weight. But we hope that the recipes we've gathered here from leading nutrition experts and our own home will at least give those striving to lose weight and adopt a healthier lifestyle a starting place for considering what a healthy meal looks like, and how much of it one should eat.

Keep in mind that sometimes difficulty losing weight can signal an underlying health condition, like an underactive thyroid. If you feel that you are already restricting your caloric intake and still can't seem to lose weight, visit the doctor for blood work. No one should suffer with a meal plan that leaves him feeling hungry. And of course one key element of any major lifestyle change, including an effort to lose weight, is patience and compassion for yourself. You won't get there overnight. But if you stick with it, you will eventually, over time. And there are many resources besides this book out there—other books, support groups, internet tools, and assistance offered by many gyms—that may also be of some assistance.

That said, we do have just a few thoughts on things that may help along the way.

The Three Diets

In *Favorite Foods from the People's Pharmacy* (2009) and *The People's Pharmacy Quick and Handy Home Remedies* (2011), which we are publishing in partnership with National Geographic, we've outlined the basics of three diets with proven health benefits: **The DASH Diet, The Low-Carb Diet**, and **The Mediterranean Diet.** Most people will lose weight if they stick to any of them. The key, of course, is to stick to them.

DASH (Dietary Approaches to Stop Hypertension) was specifically designed for people with high blood pressure. It incorporates lots of seasonings, vegetables, fruits, and whole grains, and more modest helpings of lean proteins, low-fat dairy, and nuts. You can find out more at: dashdiet.org/ or: www.nhlbi.nih.gov/health/public/heart/hbp/dash/new_dash.pdf. The researchers who put together the original study also put out a book: *The DASH* Diet for Hypertension: Lower Your Blood Pressure in 14 Days—Without Drugs*, by Thomas Moore, MD, and his colleagues (Free Press: 2001).

The Low-Carb Diet has been around for decades, popularized by Dr. Robert Atkins in the 1970s. While this approach has experienced its share of controversy over the years, more and more data indicate that a low-carbohydrate diet can be quite effective at helping people lose weight (Dansinger, et al, 2005; Foster, et al, 2003; Gardner, et al, 2007; Yancy, et al, 2004). Other benefits appear to be decreasing blood pressure and improving cholesterol, as well as helping to control blood sugar. There are any number of books available on different low-carb diets. They all share the same basic idea: that it's best to limit or eliminate simple sugars, starches, and other high-glycemic index foods, and to stick with foods like vegetables and proteins that will not cause spikes in blood sugar. Fat is not forbidden, but fruit is, at least initially. One of the contributors to this book recently co-authored a book on the low-carb diet: *The New Atkins for a New You* (Fireside: 2010) was written by Dr. Eric C. Westman with Dr. Stephen D. Phinney and Dr. Jeff S. Volek.

The Mediterranean Diet is in some ways similar to DASH in that it incorporates many fruits, vegetables, and whole grains. One of the primary ways in which it differs is in the kinds of fats and proteins it incorporates. It relies primarily on olive oil for fat, and on lots of fish, legumes, and tree nuts for protein. This diet's many health benefits are legion, and more evidence mounts daily about its ability to help protect people against diabetes and heart disease, cancer, Alzheimer's, and all sorts of other terminal conditions. Again, there are many resources available for finding out more about the Mediterranean Diet, from the website of the Mayo Clinic (http://www.mayoclinic.com/health/mediterranean-diet/ CL00011) to yet another contributor to this book, Dr. Michael Ozner, author of *The Miami Mediterranean Diet* (Cambridge House Publishing: 2005).

Green Tea

Some evidence suggests that the caffeine and catechins (a type of flavonoids) found in green tea may help with weight loss (Hursel, et al, 2009; Phung, et al, 2010; Westerterp-Plantenga, 2010). But the effects on weight loss and weight management are almost invariably described by the researchers who have conducted these studies as "modest." Furthermore, it seems that ethnicity may be a moderating factor—Caucasians are apparently somewhat less likely to experience the effects of catechins than Asians, for example (Hursel, et al, 2009).

We think green tea is wonderful, and drinking it regularly may have all sorts of other benefits, from a decreased risk of Parkinson's and Alzheimer's disease (Weinreb, et al, 2009) to cancer prevention, specifically prostate cancer (Boehm, et al, 2009), to improved cardiovascular health (Moore, et al, 2009), to stronger bones (Shen, et al, 2009). Who knows? It may even help you lose weight. If so, one reason may be that instead of reaching for another pack of crackers or cookies, you wind up reaching for your mug of green tea instead.

ONE WARNING: people being treated for multiple myeloma with a drug called bortezomib should avoid green tea.

Sugarfree Gum

There are absolutely no studies suggesting that sugarfree gum will help you lose weight, and unlike green tea, it doesn't contain any ingredients that may have this outcome. (You should be warned that if you chew too much of it, it can have a laxative effect, although this is not a good method for weight loss.) But inveterate snackers may find that chewing sugarfree gum is one way to keep them from snacking on higher-calorie treats, especially during that crucial early stage of a weight-loss program when your body and brain are trying to develop a new relationship to food and cravings for sweets may be at a high point. Just try not to overdo it: not only does nearly all sugarfree gum contain aspartame, which many people prefer to avoid, but it also contains lots of things that your body can't digest, so it can create gas, cramping, and bloating.

··· REFERENCES ···

Boehm, K., Borrelli, F., et al. "Green tea (*Camellia sinensis*) for the prevention of cancer." *Cochrane Database of Systematic Reviews* (online) 2009 Jul 8;(3): CD005004.

Clark, A., Franklin, J., et al. "Overweight and obesity—use of portion control in management." *Australian Family Physician* 2010; 39(6):407-11.

Dansinger, M. L., Gleason, J. A., et al. "Comparison of the Atkins, Ornish, Weight Watchers, and Zone Diets for weight loss and heart disease risk reduction: a randomized trial." *Journal of the American Medical Association* 2005; 293:43–53.

Foster, G. D., et al. "A randomized trial of a low-carbohydrate diet for obesity." *New England Journal of Medicine* 2003; 348:2082–2090.

Gardner, C. D., Kiazand, A., et al. "Comparison of the Atkins, Zone, Ornish, and LEARN diets for change in weight and related risk factors among overweight premenopausal women: the A to Z weight loss study: a randomized trial." *Journal of the American Medical Association* 2007; 297:969-977.

Hursel, R., Viechtbauer, W., et al. "The effects of green tea on weight loss and weight maintenance: a meta-analysis." *International Journal of Obesity* 2009; 33(9):956-61. Epub 2009 Jul 14.

King, N., Hopkins, M., et al. "Beneficial effects of exercise: Shifting the focus from body weight to other markers of health." *British Journal of Sports Medicine* 2009; 43:924-927.

MacLean, P.S., Higgins, J.A., et al. "Regular exercise attenuates the metabolic drive to regain weight after long-term weight loss." *American Journal of Physiology: Regulatory, Integrative, and Comparative Physiology* 2009; 297(3):R793-802. Epub 2009 Jul 8.

Melanson, E., Gozansky, W.S., et al. "When energy balance is maintained, exercise does not induce negative fat balance in lean sedentary, obese sedentary, or lean endurance-trained individuals." *Journal of Applied Physiology* 2009; 107:1847-1856.

Moore, R. J., Jackson, K. G., and Minihane, A. M. "Green tea (*Camellia sinensis*) catechins and vascular function." *British Journal of Nutrition* 2009; 102(12):1790-1802.

Neighmond, Patty. "Can You Be Fat and Fit? More Health Experts Say Yes." National Public Radio (npr.org) July 5, 2010.

Ozner, Michael, M.D., *The Miami Mediterranean Diet* (Cambridge House Publishing, 2005).

Phung, O.J., Baker, W.L., et al. "Effect of green tea catechins with or without caffeine on anthropometric measures: a systematic review and meta-analysis." *American Journal of Clinical Nutrition* 2010; 91(1):73-81.

Shen, C. L. Chyu, M. C., et al. "Green tea polyphenols and tai chi for bone health: Designing a placebo-controlled randomized trial." BMC *Musculoskeletal Disorders* 2009 Sept 4; 10:110.

Weinreb, O., Amit, T., et al. "Neuroprotective molecular mechanisms of (-)-epi- gallocatechin-3-gallate: A reflective outcome of its antioxidant, iron chelating and neuritogenic properties." *Genes & Nutrition* 2009 Sept 10 [Epub ahead of print]

Westerterp-Plantenga, M.S. "Green tea catechins, caffeine and body-weight regulation." *Physiology & Behavior* 2010; 100(1): 42-46. Epub 2010 Feb 13.

Westman, Eric C., M.D., with Dr. Stephen D. Phinney and Dr. Jeff S. Volek. *The New Atkins for a New You* (New York: Fireside, 2010).

Yancy, W. S., Jr., Olsen, M. K., et al. "A low-carbohydrate, ketogenic diet versus a low-fat diet to treat obesity and hyperlipidemia." *Annals of Internal Medicine* 2004; 140:769–777.

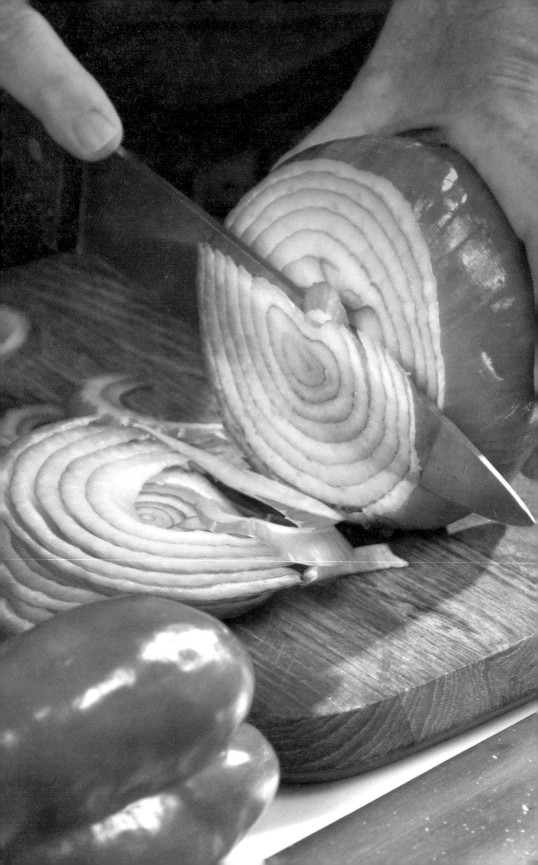

**TWO WEEKS OF
HEALTHY & DELICIOUS**

Meals & Recipes

··· SPRING & SUMMER MEALS···

··· MONDAY ···

Breakfast

Joe's Brain-Boosting Smoothie

Mid-morning snack

Small handful of almonds or walnuts (8-10 nuts)

Lunch

Spicy Fresh Tuna Salad

Dinner

Cardamom Grilled Chicken with Mango Lime Sauce
Fennel Salad

··· TUESDAY ···

Breakfast

Live & Active

Mid-morning snack

Small handful of almonds or walnuts (8-10 nuts)

Lunch

Naked Salad

Dinner

Pescado al Cilantro
Coleslaw with Mint

Dessert

Fresh Fruit Kabobs and Cinnamon Honey Dip

··· WEDNESDAY ···

Breakfast

Favorite Fish Platter

Mid-morning snack

Small piece of fruit

Lunch

Quinoa Radish Salad

Dinner

Pork & Pineapple Curry with Coconut Chutney

Dessert

A couple of squares of dark chocolate

··· THURSDAY ···

Breakfast

Mango Smoothie

Mid-morning snack

Small handful of almonds or walnuts (8-10 nuts)

Lunch

Israeli Couscous with Roasted Summer Vegetables & Nuts

Dinner

Fish Tacos with Radish & Lime
Tangy Tangerine Cress Salad

··· FRIDAY ···

Breakfast

Live & Active

Mid-morning snack

Small piece of fruit

Lunch

Fresh Mediterranean Salad

Dinner

Salmon with Fava Bean & Spring Pea Mash
Grilled Garlic Green Beans

Dessert

Cantaloupe with Lime & Mint

··· SATURDAY ···

Breakfast

Shrimp & Grits

Mid-morning snack

Small piece of fruit

Lunch

Spring Straciatella Soup
Coleslaw with Mint

Dinner

Grilled Tofu & Avocado Salad with
Blood Orange Vinaigrette

Dessert

Blueberry Cheesecake

··· SUNDAY ···

Brunch

Favorite Fish Platter

Mid-morning snack

Small piece of fruit
Small handful of almonds or walnuts (8-10 nuts)

Dinner

Lemon Roasted Chicken with Cucumber Yogurt Sauce
Veggie Dips

Dessert

Key Lime Custard

···FALL & WINTER MEALS···

···MONDAY···

Breakfast

Cholesterol-Combating Oatmeal

Mid-morning snack

Small handful of almonds or walnuts (8-10 nuts)

Lunch

Poached Eggs and Asparagus

Dinner

Horseradish Crusted Salmon with
Cranberry Catsup
Roasted Brussels Sprouts

··· TUESDAY ···

Breakfast

Anti-Inflammatory Curcumin Scramble

Mid-morning snack

Small piece of fruit

Lunch

Gypsy Soup
Kale Chips

Dinner

Chicken Adobo

Dessert

A couple of squares of dark chocolate

··· WEDNESDAY ···

Breakfast

Marigold Frittata

Mid-morning snack

Small handful of almonds or walnuts (8-10 nuts)

Lunch

Lentil and Roasted Bell Pepper Salad

Dinner

Penne with Broccoli and Sundried Tomato

Dessert

Poached Pears

··· THURSDAY ···

Breakfast

Cinnamon-Almond Oatmeal

Mid-morning snack

Small piece of fruit

Lunch

Cauliflower and Red Pepper Quiche

Dinner

Cannellini, Collard & Sausage Stew
Roasted Garlic

··· FRIDAY ···

Breakfast

Poached Eggs with Spinach

Mid-morning snack

Small piece of fruit

Lunch

Curry Soup

Dinner

Lentil Nut Loaf with Red Pepper Sauce
Farmer's Market Saag

Dessert

A couple of squares of dark chocolate

··· SATURDAY ···

Breakfast

Cholesterol-Combating Oatmeal

Mid-morning snack

Small handful of almonds or walnuts (8-10 nuts)

Lunch

Bitter Melon Stir Fry

Dinner

Leek & Sweet Onion Frittata
Curried Sweet Potato Fries

Dessert

Three-Layer Mousse

··· SUNDAY ···

Breakfast

Anti-Inflammatory Scramble

Mid-morning snack

Small handful of almonds or walnuts (8-10 nuts)

Lunch

Butternut Squash and Apple Soup
Wheat Berry Salad

Dinner

Cancer-Fighting Cabbage Curry

Dessert

Roasted Peaches

··· RECIPES ···

··· BREAKFAST ···

Anti-Inflammatory Curcumin Scramble

4 large eggs (if you prefer, substitute two egg whites
  for one of the eggs)
Pinch salt and ground black pepper
1 teaspoon turmeric powder (a source of curcumin)
2 tablespoons milk or water
  (milk will make the eggs denser and creamier;
  water, fluffier and lighter)
1 tablespoon olive or grape seed oil
½ teaspoon grated Parmesan
Sprinkling of chopped chives

In a medium-sized mixing bowl, use a fork to mix eggs, salt, pepper, and powdered turmeric. (Be very careful with the turmeric: it will dye everything it touches a bright, summery yellow.)

Add olive or grape seed oil to a large sauté pan or skillet, and set your burner to medium-low heat. While the oil is heating, stir milk or water into your egg mixture. When oil is hot, pour egg mixture into pan or skillet. Let eggs set for 15-20 seconds before gently scrambling with a wooden spatula. Add Parmesan. Let set for another 15 seconds, and gently scramble again. Repeat until eggs are cooked.

Serve, and garnish with chives. Makes two servings.

Cholesterol-Combating Oatmeal

1 cup soy milk
¼ cup steel-cut oats
1 teaspoon ground cinnamon
Pinch salt
½ cup egg whites
¼ cup dried fruit (we like currants,
    raisins, and cherries), or 2/3 cup fresh fruit
2 tablespoons ground flaxseed
⅓ cup chopped walnuts or almonds
2 teaspoons honey, agave nectar, maple syrup,
    or sugar substitute (optional)

Bring soy milk to a boil in a medium saucepan. (We recommend using a lid so that no milk escapes as it begins to boil.)

Add oats, cinnamon, and salt. Stir and reduce heat to a simmer. Continue stirring while adding the egg whites, then cook uncovered over low heat for about 10 minutes, stirring occasionally.

Add fruit, flaxseed, and nuts, and cook until oats are tender, approximately 10-15 minutes more.

Top each serving with sweetener to taste, if desired. Makes two generous helpings.

Cinnamon-Almond Oatmeal

I cup soy or rice milk
⅔ cup rolled oats
Pinch salt (optional)
2 tablespoons ground flaxseed
⅓ cup chopped almonds
I teaspoon ground cinnamon
Sugar substitute to taste (optional)

Bring soy or rice milk to a boil in a medium saucepan. (We recommend using a lid so that no milk escapes as it begins to boil.) Add oats and salt. Stir and reduce heat to a simmer. Cook uncovered over low heat for about two to three minutes, stirring occasionally. Add flaxseed, and cook until oats are tender, approximately five minutes more.

Top each serving with cinnamon, almonds, and sweetener to taste, if desired. Makes two generous helpings.

Favorite Fish Platter

½ pound smoked fish (for breakfast,
    we especially like trout or salmon)
2 poached or hard-boiled eggs
1 cup mixed greens and arugula
¼ of a red onion, thinly sliced
Several slices avocado
Several slices cucumber

Dressing for greens:
1 teaspoon olive oil
1 teaspoon lemon juice
1 teaspoon Dijon mustard
Pinch salt and pepper

Garnish:
1 or 2 teaspoons drained capers
Lemon wedges

To make the dressing for the greens, whisk the olive oil, lemon juice, mustard, and salt and pepper in the bottom of a medium bowl with a fork. (Mix in chopped chives or scallions as well, if you like.) Add arugula and greens to the bowl, and mix until greens are coated with dressing.

Arrange greens on two plates. Top with avocado, red onion, and cucumber. Add one egg and ¼ pound of fish to each plate. Garnish with capers and lemon wedge. Makes two servings.

This is a lovely weekend brunch that should keep you filled up until mid-afternoon.

Joe's Brain-Boosting Smoothie

1 teaspoon fish oil
1 frozen banana
1 cup fresh or frozen mixed berries
If using fresh berries: 1 cup crushed ice
¾ cup plain yogurt
½ cup pomegranate or cherry juice
½ cup pasteurized egg whites
  (or roughly 4 eggs' worth)
4 tablespoons whey powder
2 tablespoons ground flaxseed

Add all ingredients to a blender. Puree until smooth. You may need to scrape down the sides once or twice with a spatula to ensure that the mixture is evenly blended. Pour into tall glasses and enjoy right away, or chill in the refrigerator overnight. Makes two generous servings.

Live & Active

½ cup low-fat Greek or other yogurt
2-3 drops vanilla extract (optional)
½ cup fresh seasonal fruit
¼ cup walnuts or almonds, chopped
1 tablespoon wheat germ
2 teaspoons ground flaxseed
1 teaspoon honey, agave nectar, maple sugar,
  jam, or sugar substitute (optional)

Select a yogurt with live and active cultures (it should say on the container). If using the vanilla extract, fold it into the yogurt. Top with the remaining ingredients and enjoy. Makes a very hearty serving for one.

Mango Smoothie

Contributed by Jeffrey Blumberg, PhD
and Helen Rasmussen, PhD, RD, FADA.

The recipe below is based on one used in a clinical trial created
at the Human Nutrition Research Center on Aging.

20 ounces unsweetened apple juice
2 ½ cups fresh or frozen strawberries
1 ¾ cups frozen mango pieces
2 cups mashed bananas

Place the apple juice and strawberries in a blender. Cover and blend on high until smooth. Add half of the mango pieces. Cover and blend on high for approximately one minute. Add the remaining mango pieces. Cover and blend on high for approximately 30 seconds, then add the bananas and blend for another 30 seconds. Makes eight servings.

Here is Dr. Blumberg and Dr. Rasmussen's story of how this recipe came to be:

"This recipe was created for two dietary studies. One study was targeted to increasing the intake of the carotenoids beta-carotene and lutein. Carotenoids are antioxidants that provide many fruits and vegetables with their orange, red, or yellow colors.

"The other study was designed to promote an alkaline-producing diet (producing a slightly higher pH of the blood) and contrast it with an acid-producing diet. Diets rich in meat and cereals produce a lower blood pH (more acidic) while more fruit and vegetables raise the pH. Alkaline diets may help retain bone mineral density and reduce the risk for osteoporosis and bone fracture.

"At the end of these studies, many of the volunteers requested the recipe for this mango smoothie."

Marigold Frittata

Contributed by Jeffrey Blumberg, PhD
and Helen Rasmussen, PhD, RD, FADA.

The recipe below is based on one used in a clinical trial created
at the Human Nutrition Research Center on Aging.

4 eggs
1 tablespoon water, plus additional water
   for water bath
½ cup sliced mushrooms
1 tablespoon grated Parmesan cheese
¼ cup finely chopped onion
3 tablespoons olive oil, plus additional oil
   for greasing casserole dish
Salt and pepper to taste

Preheat oven to 350 degrees. Grease a small casserole dish. Add a small amount of water to a larger Pyrex dish. (This will serve as the water bath for cooking the frittata.)

Sauté the onion in olive oil for two to three minutes. Add mushrooms, and sauté for an additional 10 minutes. Transfer the onions and mushrooms to the casserole dish. Crack eggs into a large mixing bowl, and whisk together with the tablespoon of water. Pour the eggs into the casserole dish, and stir them into the vegetables. Sprinkle Parmesan over the mixture. Place the casserole dish into the water bath, and transfer both dishes to the oven. Cook uncovered for 15 minutes.

The frittata is done when a fork inserted into the middle comes out clean. Makes two servings.

Here is Dr. Blumberg and Dr. Rasmussen's story of how this recipe came to be:

"This egg dish was created for a study measuring the ability of the carotenoid lutein to be absorbed from food into the blood. Lutein is an antioxidant found in high concentrations in the retina where it has been associated with a reduced risk of age-related macular degeneration, the leading cause of blindness in older adults. Lutein is also found in high concentrations in the brain, where it may act to support cognitive function.

"The dish was named the marigold frittata because the whole eggs that were used in the study were made lutein-rich by feeding yellow marigold petals, a good source of lutein, to the chickens that produced them."

Poached Eggs with Spinach

4 poached eggs
1 large bunch of fresh spinach,
    washed and dried, or 1 10-ounce package
    of frozen spinach, thawed and pressed dry
1 tablespoon grape seed or olive oil
1 clove garlic, minced or pressed
1 tablespoon fresh thyme, chopped (optional)
1 teaspoon crushed hot pepper flakes (optional)
Salt and freshly ground pepper to taste

In a medium-sized skillet, heat the oil over medium heat, lightly sauté the garlic, then add the spinach. Cook until just wilted.

Divide the cooked spinach onto two plates, top with two poached eggs, and garnish with thyme and hot pepper flakes, if desired. Add salt and pepper to taste. Makes two servings.

Shrimp & Grits

Cheese Grits:
½ cup stone-ground grits
2 cups water
Salt to taste
1 tablespoon butter
Freshly ground white and black pepper
Half of a fresh jalapeño, de-seeded,
    ribbed, and chopped
¼ cup sharp Cheddar, grated

Shrimp:
1 tablespoon grape seed or olive oil
¾ pound fresh shrimp, peeled
    and deveined
1 cup sliced mushrooms
½ cup scallions, sliced
1 small clove garlic, minced or pressed
1 teaspoon lemon juice
Drizzle truffle oil (optional)

To prepare the grits: soak the grits in a large bowl of cold water for ten minutes, skim off the chaff, and drain the grits. Bring the two cups of water to boil and stir in the grits and a pinch of salt. Turn the heat down to low and let the grits simmer, stirring regularly, until cooked (about 35 to 40 minutes). Remove from the heat and stir in the remaining ingredients for the grits.

To prepare the shrimp: heat the oil in a skillet over medium-high. When the oil is hot but not yet smoking, add the shrimp. Sauté until they start to become opaque and add the mushrooms, stirring often. Sauté until the shrimp are pink and the mushrooms are cooked, about three or four minutes more, and add the garlic and scallions. Stir several times and then serve while both shrimp and grits are still hot.

Each serving should receive about half a cup of grits and be topped with half a portion of the shrimp. Squeeze a bit of lemon juice and drizzle a few drops of truffle oil over each dish. Makes two servings.

··· MAIN DISHES ···

Bitter Melon Stir Fry

2 bitter melons, prepared
2 tablespoons of grape seed oil
Half of an onion, diced
   (or substitute 2 chopped scallions)
1 clove garlic, minced or pressed
2 tablespoons red wine vinegar
1 tablespoon soy sauce
1 tablespoon ginger, peeled
   and grated (optional)
½ teaspoon chili flakes (optional)

To prepare bitter melon: if you're looking to remove as much of the bitter flavor as possible, you may want to deseed and parboil the melons before sautéing them. Chop off both ends of the melon and slice it lengthwise. Then scoop out the seeds and the white, fibrous flesh inside with a spoon. Slice the melon (leaving the skin on) into quarter-inch pieces. Then bring water to boil in a large pot and parboil the melon slices for about five minutes. You can also leave the seeds in, if you prefer, and soak the melon in room-temperature salted water for 30 minutes rather than parboiling. If you go this route, you'll need to sauté the slices for slightly longer.

To prepare the stir fry: heat the grape seed oil in a large skillet, wok or sauté pan on medium heat. Sauté the onions until translucent (three to four minutes). Add the garlic, and stir frequently to prevent from burning. Add the chili flakes and ginger, if using. Then add the prepared bitter melon slices, and sauté for two minutes or so. Add the vinegar and soy sauce, and sauté for another two minutes, or until the bitter melon is tender. Makes two servings.

For protein, you can add tofu, beef, pork, or egg to the stir fry before the bitter melon slices if you like.

Butternut Squash and Apple Soup

4 pounds butternut squash, peeled,
   seeded, and cut lengthwise
3 tablespoons cooking oil
   (walnut, grape seed, and olive all work well)
1 medium-sized onion, chopped finely
3 medium-sized apples, cored and
   sliced thinly (Braeburn work well)
2 cups apple juice or cider
1 tablespoon cider vinegar
8 cups low-sodium chicken broth
   or stock
1½ tablespoons sea salt
Freshly ground black pepper
6 ounces sharp cheddar (optional)
6 ounces nuts for garnish (toasted walnuts,
   pistachios, or pumpkin seeds all work well)

Preheat the oven to 350 degrees. Place the squash sliced side down in a large oven-safe baking dish, and fill the dish with about two cups of water. Roast the butternut squash until tender (roughly 35 to 45 minutes).

In a large stock pot, heat the oil and sauté the onion until translucent (about 8 or 10 minutes). Add most of the apple slices (reserve some for garnish), and sauté for another five or six minutes, until apple is soft. Add the apple juice or cider and bring to a boil. Reduce the heat and let simmer until about half of the liquid has evaporated.

When the squash has cooled enough to handle, cut it into small pieces and add it to the soup. Add the cider vinegar, chicken broth, salt, and pepper, and again bring to a boil. Reduce the heat to a simmer, and let cook until the squash, apple, and onions are quite soft (about 20 minutes).

In batches, puree the soup in a blender. Adjust seasoning to taste. Serve warm, and garnish each bowl with several slices of apple, a small chunk of cheddar cheese, and several toasted nuts. Makes six servings.

Cancer-Fighting Cabbage Curry

2 tablespoons walnut oil
¼ cup walnuts, chopped
1 teaspoon black mustard seeds
¾ cup minced leek
1 teaspoon turmeric
½ teaspoon curry powder
6 stalks of celery, coarsely chopped
½ small head red cabbage,
   coarsely chopped (about 3 cups)
⅔ cup chicken or vegetable broth
Salt and freshly ground black pepper to taste
½ cup minced parsley
½ pound tofu (a little more than half of
   an average block), cut into 2-inch by 1-inch pieces
½ cup rice vinegar

Heat the walnut oil at medium heat in a large skillet. Sauté the walnuts, remove and reserve. Add the black mustard seeds, and when they begin to pop, add the leeks. Sauté until they are soft, then add the turmeric and curry powder. Stir for about 30 seconds, then add the celery. Sauté for a few minutes, then add cabbage. Turn the heat to low, add the broth, cover, and let simmer for about 15 minutes.

When the cabbage is tender, add salt and black pepper to taste. Stir in the parsley. Slide the vegetables aside to make room in the center of the pan, then add the tofu. Stir the tofu and vegetables for another 6 to 8 minutes, until the liquid has evaporated.

Add the vinegar, top the dish with the walnuts, and serve. Makes four servings.

This dish contains apigenin (from the celery and the parsley), quercetin (from the leeks), genistein (from the tofu), isothiocyanate (from the cabbage), and walnut flavonoids. These phytonutrients have been shown to be active against prostate cancer cells in laboratory tests.

Cannellini, Collard, and Sausage Stew

2 bunches fresh collards, ribs and stems removed
and sliced into half-inch pieces
3 tablespoons olive or grape seed oil
1 large onion, peeled and diced
1½ teaspoons Kosher salt
Freshly ground black pepper to taste
½ teaspoon crushed hot pepper flakes (optional)
1 tablespoon red wine vinegar
2 cans cannellini (white) beans, rinsed
1 clove garlic, minced or pressed
4 fresh lean sausages (lamb works well)

To prepare the collards: heat two tablespoons of the oil in a large stock pot. When hot, sauté half of the onion until translucent. Add the salt, pepper, and hot pepper flakes, then add the collards and sauté briefly. Add enough water to cover the collards and bring to a boil. Reduce the heat to a simmer and cook for at least an hour, up to an hour and a half. (The goal is for the collards to be quite tender, but not mushy.) If the water cooks away, add more in small amounts as necessary, stirring often.

When collards are about 20 minutes from being done, heat the oil in a large skillet until hot but not smoking, and sauté the remaining onion and garlic for several minutes. Add the sausages, and cook over medium heat for about seven or eight minutes, or until they're very browned on one side. Then turn them over and cook for an additional six or seven minutes, or until browned on the other side.

Deglaze the pan with the vinegar. Add the cannellini beans and collards with some of their cooking liquid, and cook for an additional five or so minutes. Adjust seasoning to taste. Makes four servings.

Cardamom Grilled Chicken with Mango Lime Sauce

Contributed by Mark Liponis, MD,
author of UltraLongevity: The Seven-Step Program for
a Younger, Healthier You, *from which this recipe is taken.*

Spice mix:
3 tablespoons cardamom
1 tablespoon black pepper
1 tablespoon salt
1 teaspoon cinnamon
¼ teaspoon cayenne pepper

Six 4-ounce skinless chicken breasts,
   boned and defatted

Sauce:
1 mango, cleaned and diced
½ cup lime juice
2 tablespoons olive oil
1 tablespoon minced ginger
½ cup nonfat plain yogurt
½ teaspoon salt
1 tablespoon diced jalapeño
1 tablespoon chopped cilantro

Prepare coals for grilling or preheat broiler. In a small bowl, combine ingredients for spice mix. Lightly pound chicken breasts to flatten. Dust each with about 1 teaspoon spice mix. Store remaining spice mix in an airtight container for future use.

Grill chicken for three to five minutes on each side, or until juices run clear when piercedwith a fork.

Combine all ingredients for sauce in a blender, except for jalapeño and cilantro. Puree until smooth. Pour into a bowl, add jalapeño and cilantro, and gently stir.

Serve one chicken breast with ¼ cup sauce. Makes six servings.

Chicken Adobo

6 pieces of chicken
1 cup soy sauce
1 cup white vinegar
1 six-inch piece of fresh ginger root,
   peeled and sliced thin
1 tablespoon garlic, minced
2 tablespoons brown sugar

Preheat the oven to 350 degrees. Combine all of the ingredients in a casserole dish, making sure that the chicken pieces are well covered in sauce.

Bake for just over an hour and serve hot. Makes six servings.

Crustless Cauliflower and Red Pepper Quiche
Contributed by Eric C. Westman, MD, MHS

1 teaspoon olive oil, plus more for pie plate
½ small onion, finely chopped
½ red bell pepper, diced
4 large eggs
½ cup heavy cream
1 cup water
1 cup grated Monterey Jack cheese, divided
¼ teaspoon dried thyme
¼ teaspoon dried oregano
¼ teaspoon chopped dried rosemary
½ teaspoon salt
¼ teaspoon pepper
1 small head cauliflower, cut into florets,
   stems peeled and cut 1/3-inch thick
   (substitute broccoli, if you prefer)

Heat oven to 375 degrees. Brush a 9- or 10-inch pie plate with olive oil. Heat oil in a small skillet over medium-high heat. Add onion and red pepper and cook until softened, about three minutes. Transfer to a medium bowl and let cool. Add eggs to onion and lightly beat. Whisk in cream, water, ½ cup cheese, herbs, salt and pepper to blend.

Cover bottom of pie plate with cauliflower or broccoli. Cover with cream mixture and sprinkle with remaining ½ cup cheese. Bake until a knife inserted in middle comes out clean and quiche is golden brown, 50 to 60 minutes. Makes six servings.

Dr. Westman suggests: "This makes a great low-carb breakfast, or serve it with a tossed salad for lunch."

Curry Soup

⅓ cup brown basmati rice
2 cups water
1 tablespoon safflower oil
1 cup red onion, diced
2 celery stalks, diced
2 carrots, peeled and diced
2 cloves garlic, pressed
½ teaspoon curry powder
1 teaspoon turmeric
¼ teaspoon fresh ground black pepper
3 cups vegetable broth
¾ cup diced tofu
12 ounces coconut water or clear coconut juice
Lime wedges for garnish

Place the rice in the 2 cups of water and set to simmer before chopping the vegetables.

In a saucepan, heat the safflower oil and sauté the garlic and vegetables. Once the vegetables soften, lower the heat, and stir in the curry powder, turmeric, and pepper. After about 1 minute, add the broth, and simmer the vegetable mixture for an additional 15 or so minutes.

Add the diced tofu, and cook for several minutes, stirring occasionally. While the tofu is simmering, strain the rice, and then add it and the coconut water to the mixture.

Adjust the salt to taste. Garnish each bowl with a wedge of lime. Makes four servings.

Fish Tacos with Radish and Lime

Fish Marinade:
4 fillets of very fresh, firm, white-fleshed fish:
   cod, haddock, or halibut work well
1 cup chopped red onion
½ cup fresh chopped cilantro, de-stemmed
¼ cup olive oil
½ teaspoon salt
½ teaspoon freshly ground black pepper
¼ teaspoon chipotle powder or hot sauce

Tacos:
8 small soft flour tortillas
2 medium-sized ripe avocados, sliced
2 fresh jalapeños, seeded, ribbed, and sliced
6 medium radishes, chopped
4 limes, 2 sliced into wedges

Chipotle aioli:
½ cup light mayonnaise
1 clove garlic, minced or pressed
1 teaspoon lime juice
1 teaspoon Dijon mustard

½ to I teaspoon chipotle powder
or hot sauce
Pinch salt and pepper

To prepare fish: mix onion, cilantro, olive oil, salt, pepper, and chipotle powder in a medium-sized bowl. Transfer about half of the mixture to a fairly shallow dish in order to marinade the fish fillets. Place the fillets over the mixture, and then spoon the remaining marinade over them. Put dish into the fridge for 30 minutes. Flip fillets over, and return to the fridge to marinate for another 20-30 minutes.

While the fish is marinating, mix together the ingredients for the aioli and set aside. (It's best if served at room temperature, but don't leave out for more than 20 to 30 minutes.)

Grease grill grate of either outdoor barbeque or indoor grilling pan, and heat to medium-high heat. Cook fillets until white and flaky (about 3 to 5 minutes per side, depending upon the thickness of the fish). Sprinkle each cooked fillet with a liberal amount of squeezed lime juice (roughly half a lime).

Heat flour tortillas by wrapping them in aluminum foil and placing them on the grill for a couple of minutes while fish are cooking.

Prepare each taco with half of a grilled fish fillet, two slices of avocado, a sprinkling of chopped radishes and sliced jalapeños, and a small dollop (roughly 1 tablespoon) of chipotle aioli. Garnish the plate with a lime wedge. Makes eight small tortillas and serves four.

Fresh Mediterranean Salad

2 cups washed and dried mixed greens
Half of a large red pepper, chopped
Half a pint of grape or cherry tomatoes,
   halved or quartered
Half of a medium-sized cucumber, diced
Half of a ripe avocado, diced
2 hardboiled eggs, peeled and chopped
¼ cup feta, crumbled
¼ cup walnuts, toasted
1 tablespoon extra-virgin olive oil
1 tablespoon lemon juice
1 tablespoon Dijon
Pinch salt and freshly ground black pepper

Whisk together the olive oil, lemon juice, Dijon, and pinch of salt and freshly ground pepper in a large bowl. Add the greens and toss until the leaves are coated in a thin film of dressing. Add the remaining ingredients and toss. Makes two servings.

Variations include: adding half of a 12-ounce can of garbanzo beans (chickpeas), drained and rinsed; or adding a can of canned, light tuna (not albacore) that has been packed in oil. Drain the oil and flake into the salad with a fork.

Grilled Tofu & Avocado Salad with Blood Orange Vinaigrette

Tofu:
- 1 14-ounce block of extra-firm tofu, drained and sliced crosswise into 8 pieces
- 4 tablespoons olive oil
- 2 tablespoons low-sodium soy sauce
- 2 tablespoons red wine vinegar
- 2 teaspoons sesame oil
- 3 cloves garlic, minced or pressed
- 2 scallions, chopped finely
- 2 teaspoons ginger, peeled and grated or finely diced
- ½ teaspoon crushed hot pepper flakes (optional)
- Pinch salt and freshly ground black pepper

Vinaigrette:
- 2 tablespoons freshly squeezed blood orange juice (can substitute grapefruit juice)
- 1 tablespoon lemon juice
- 1 tablespoon Dijon
- 1 tablespoon extra-virgin olive oil
- Salt and pepper to taste

Salad:
- 10 ounces mixed greens, washed and dried
- 2 ripe avocados, sliced
- 1 yellow or orange bell pepper, sliced thin
- ½ cup fresh cilantro, washed, dried, and chopped

To prepare the tofu: In a liquid measuring cup (or something else that will easily pour), whisk together the olive oil, soy sauce, red wine vinegar, sesame oil, garlic, scallions, and ginger. Place the pieces of tofu in a small, shallow glass dish, and pour the marinade over them. After 30 minutes, turn the pieces of tofu over in the marinade, spoon any extra sauce over them, and let marinade for at least another 20 minutes while the indoor or outdoor grill is heating. (Can also be left covered overnight in the fridge.)

Grill tofu slices until grill marks appear, flipping once—three to four minutes per side. (If you prefer, you can pan sear the tofu instead. Heat about one tablespoon of grape seed oil in a large skillet or sauté pan over medium-high heat until hot but not smoking. When you place the tofu in the skillet, it should sizzle. Cook for roughly three minutes, until tofu has browned on one side, and then flip to the other side and cook for an additional three minutes.)

To prepare the vinaigrette: Whisk all vinaigrette ingredients with a fork in the bottom of a large bowl.

Add the greens to the bowl a bit at a time, tossing as you go, until all the greens are evenly coated with the dressing. Divide the greens onto three plates, and top each serving with two to three pieces of grilled tofu, several slices avocado and yellow pepper, and cilantro for garnish. Makes three servings.

Gypsy Soup

Contributed by Christopher Gardner, PhD,
who has adapted the following recipe from one by
Mollie Katzen in the original Moosewood Cookbook.

4 tablespoons olive oil

2 medium onions, chopped

4 cloves garlic, pressed, crushed, or chopped

2 teaspoons paprika

1 teaspoon turmeric

1 teaspoon basil

¼ teaspoon cinnamon

¼ teaspoon cayenne

1 bay leaf

3 cups sweet potatoes, peeled and chopped

3 cups low sodium vegetable stock

16 ounces of tomatoes, chopped, canned
   or fresh (2 medium tomatoes if in season)

1 cup frozen peas (or fresh if in season)

15 ounces of garbanzo beans (chickpeas),
   canned (or from dried beans if preferred)

8 ounces tempeh, chopped into ½-inch cubes

1 tablespoon tamari

In a large soup pot, sauté onions and garlic in olive oil over medium heat until the onions are translucent (about four minutes). Add the spices and herbs and stir in for one minute. Add the sweet potatoes and vegetable stock, bring to a boil, and allow to simmer for fifteen minutes. Add the remaining ingredients, return to a boil, and simmer for an additional ten minutes (or until vegetables are tender).

Here are some of Dr. Gardner's thoughts on Mollie Katzen's *Gypsy Soup*:

"If I were asked to pick my favorite most healthful and delicious dish, something that has been my most frequently enjoyed staple of the last 30 years, it would be my version of Gypsy Soup that I first found in Mollie Katzen's *Moosewood Cookbook.*

"I make this recipe year-round, including times of the year when tomatoes and peas are not in season. This never stops me, as I am fine using canned tomatoes and frozen peas. It's also great to use dried garbanzo beans and cook them ahead of time, but I tend to use canned because there are so many good options available. I try to choose organic ingredients whenever possible, and as-local-as-possible ingredients for the fresh vegetables.

"You can use more vegetable stock if you prefer it more soupy, less if you prefer it more like a vegetable stew. Plenty of room for additional vegetables, including celery, roasted red bell peppers, carrots, and corn.

"This tends to be a quick recipe, although perhaps that is partly due to the fact that I make it so often. The turmeric, in particular, gives the dish a great color and aroma that make it tantalizing. This spicy dish is hearty and filling, and I usually make a double batch so I can serve some that day, put some away in the refrigerator for later in the week, and freeze some for a week when I am pinched for time (it is still quite tasty and holds up well to freezing and thawing)."

Horseradish Crusted Salmon with Cranberry Catsup

Contributed by Mark Liponis, MD,
author of UltraLongevity: The Seven-Step Program for a
Younger, Healthier You, *from which this recipe is taken.*

⅓ cup all-purpose flour
1 teaspoon salt
1 whole egg, beaten
1 tablespoon white vinegar
1 cup fresh, finely grated horseradish
4 four-ounce salmon fillets
1 teaspoon olive oil

Cranberry Dill Catsup:
¾ cup fresh or frozen cranberries
½ cup apple cider
2 teaspoons minced shallots
Pinch salt
2 teaspoons granulated sugar
2 teaspoons fresh, chopped dill

In a shallow bowl, combine flour and salt and mix well. In a separate bowl, combine egg and vinegar, and beat until combined. Spread horseradish in a medium shallow bowl. Dip salmon fillet in flour mixture, then egg mixture, and then grated horseradish. Repeat for remaining fillets.

Heat a sauté pan with olive oil, and sauté salmon over medium heat until cooked through and golden brown, about three to five minutes on each side.

In a blender, combine cranberries, apple cider, shallots, salt and sugar, and puree until smooth. Stir in chopped dill. Serve two ounces cranberry dill catsup with each salmon fillet.

Makes four servings.

Israeli Couscous with
Roasted Summer Vegetables & Nuts

1 medium-sized zucchini, chopped
½ of 1 medium-sized eggplant, chopped
½ of a bunch of asparagus, chopped and ends removed
1 red and 1 yellow pepper, chopped
½ red onion, chopped
½ pint grape or cherry tomatoes, halved or quartered
3 tablespoons extra-virgin olive oil
2 teaspoons Kosher salt
1 cup Israeli couscous
1 ½ cups low-sodium chicken broth
1 clove garlic, minced
1 tablespoon lemon juice
¼ cup basil, chopped
½ cup feta, crumbled
½ cup nuts, toasted (pine nuts or almonds work well)
Freshly ground black pepper

Preheat oven to 400 degrees.

To prepare roasted vegetables: arrange zucchini and eggplant pieces on a baking sheet and sprinkle with one tablespoon of the olive oil and a pinch of salt and pepper. Place baking sheet on a center rack in the oven, and let roast for about 15 minutes.

Remove the baking sheet from the oven, and arrange bell pepper and onion pieces on it. Drizzle with half a tablespoon of the olive oil and a bit more of the salt and pepper. Return to the center rack of the oven and roast for an additional 10 minutes.

Remove the baking sheet from the oven and add the tomatoes. Drizzle on an additional half tablespoon of olive oil and return the baking sheet to the oven for a final five minutes, or until all vegetables are tender. Remove the baking sheet from the oven and let the vegetables cool to room temperature.

To prepare Israeli couscous: bring the chicken broth to a boil. Stir in the couscous, reduce heat to a simmer, and then cook covered for about 15 minutes, or until the couscous has absorbed all of the broth. Remove from heat.

To prepare salad: in a large bowl, whisk together the garlic, lemon juice, the remaining tablespoon of olive oil, one teaspoon of salt, and freshly ground pepper. Add the couscous and toss. Add the roasted vegetables and toss. Serve, topping each serving with nuts, feta, and basil. Makes three servings.

Leek and Sweet Onion Frittata

1 tablespoon grape seed or extra-virgin olive oil,
  plus more for greasing skillet
1 medium-sized leek, thinly sliced
  (only pale green and white parts)
1 cup sweet onion, thinly sliced crosswise
1 clove garlic, minced or pressed
1 teaspoon brown sugar or sugar substitute (optional)
½ teaspoon red wine vinegar (optional)
6 large eggs
½ cup pasteurized egg whites
  (or roughly 4 eggs' worth)
2 tablespoons milk or water (milk will make the
  eggs denser and creamier; water, fluffier and lighter)
½ teaspoon salt
½ teaspoon freshly ground black pepper
¼ cup freshly grated Parmesan

Preheat the broiler and grease a medium-sized skillet or oven-safe sauté pan. Set aside.

If you'd like to caramelize the onions and leeks, heat oil in a large skillet or sauté pan over medium-high heat until it's hot but not smoking. Add the onion and leek (they should sizzle but not pop), as well as the sugar and a pinch of salt. Turn the heat down to medium-low, and stir frequently until the onion and leek are golden brown (about 20 minutes). Deglaze the pan with the vinegar, and continue to stir until the liquid has evaporated.

If you'd prefer simply to sauté the onion and leek, you can skip the sugar and the vinegar for deglazing, and cook for a much shorter period of time (8 to 10 minutes, or until the vegetables are tender).

Sauté garlic in your medium-sized skillet on medium heat. Once your vegetables are caramelized or sautéed, transfer them to the medium skillet as well, and turn the burner to low.

In a large bowl, whisk together the eggs and egg whites, milk or water, salt, and pepper. Pour the mixture into the medium-sized skillet with the vegetables, and turn the heat to medium-low. Fold gently to combine. Cook until the eggs are nearly set (about 10 to 12 minutes). Sprinkle grated Parmesan over the mixture, and place in the oven to broil until the top of the frittata is golden brown (about 3 to 5 minutes). Cut into wedges and serve. Makes four generous servings.

Lemon Roasted Chicken with Cucumber Yogurt Sauce

Chicken:
¾ cup kosher salt
2 quarts water
I whole chicken, rinsed and patted dry,
   giblets removed and discarded, and
   trimmed of any extra fat
Freshly ground black pepper
2 lemons: I quartered, I sliced
   (the first for roasting in the cavity of the bird,
   the second for garnish)
2 large cloves garlic, peeled and crushed
¼ cup extra-virgin olive oil, plus oil
   for greasing roasting pan
¾ cup lemon juice (about 4 to 6 lemons' worth)
I½ cups low-sodium chicken broth
I teaspoon minced fresh thyme (optional)

Sauce:
I large cucumber, peeled, seeded, and diced
Pinch salt
¾ cup low-fat Greek yogurt, drained
I small clove garlic, pressed
I tablespoon extra-virgin olive oil
I tablespoon lemon juice
   (can substitute red wine vinegar)
Pinch dried cayenne
¼ teaspoon freshly ground black pepper
I teaspoon chopped mint

To prepare chicken: in a very large pot, dissolve salt in water and brine chicken for about an hour in the refrigerator. (You can skip this step if in a hurry, although it does make for a very tasty bird.)

Remove the chicken from its brining bath, rinse very well, and pat dry. Rub all over with freshly ground pepper.

Set the oven to 375 degrees. If you have a V-rack, place it in a roasting pan. (If you don't, just use the roasting pan and its rack.) Grease with some oil to keep your bird from sticking.

Stuff the quartered lemon and garlic cloves inside the bird, and seal the cavity with a small skewer or twine. Before placing chicken breast-side down on the V-rack or roasting pan, rub the breast side with a tablespoon of the olive oil. Then, once it's situated on the rack, rub an additional tablespoon of olive oil on the back of the bird. Place roasting pan near the middle rack of the oven.

Roast the chicken for 40 minutes. Remove the pan from the oven and increase the heat to 450 degrees. Flip the chicken to its other side, add a cup of the broth to the roasting pan, and return to the oven. Start cucumber yogurt sauce (instructions below). Roast for about another 40 minutes, basting once. When a meat thermometer reads 170 in the thickest part of the chicken's thigh, remove chicken from oven and let cool on a carving board while making the lemon gravy.

Turn the heat off in the oven and place the roasting pan over two burners on the stove. Remove the rack, and skim the fat from the drippings off the liquid. Turn to high heat, add the remaining ½ cup of chicken broth, and while the liquid is simmering, use a wooden spoon to scrape the brown bits from the bottom of the roasting pan. Let it reduce for four or five minutes, then remove from heat while finishing the cucumber yogurt sauce. Once the cucumber yogurt sauce is prepared (or after about 10 minutes), whisk the remaining two tablespoons of olive oil into the gravy, along with the lemon juice and thyme.

Discard the lemons and garlic from the chicken cavity and carve the chicken. Pour the lemon gravy over each serving, then dollop with about ¼ cup of cucumber yogurt sauce (see next page) and garnish with lemon slices. Makes four servings.

To prepare cucumber yogurt sauce: Toss cucumber and salt in a bowl and set aside for about 20 minutes. (Do this step while the chicken is brining or roasting, or prepare the cucumber yogurt sauce up to a day ahead. It can be refrigerated, covered, overnight.) Pour fluid off of the cucumber, then mix well with the other ingredients. Refrigerate until ready to serve.

Lentil and Roasted Bell Pepper Salad
Contributed by Christopher Gardner, PhD

Salad:
1 ½ cups dry lentils
½ cup of diced onion, yellow or red
2 cloves garlic, pressed or very finely minced
1 cup diced carrot
¼ teaspoon salt
1 bay leaf
6 cups vegetable stock (or water)
2 cups roasted bell peppers (red and yellow preferred), chopped
1 tablespoon chopped mint
3 tablespoons chopped cilantro

Lemon Vinaigrette:
4 tablespoons lemon juice
1 tablespoon minced lemon peel (optional, easy if you have a lemon peeler)
2 tablespoons red wine vinegar
2 cloves garlic, pressed or very finely minced
¼ teaspoon paprika
Pinch cayenne
6 ounces olive oil

6 ounces crumbled feta cheese
(leave off for vegan option)
Pepper, to taste
8-12 cups loose mixed salad greens

Add the dry lentils, onion, garlic, carrot, salt, bay leaf, and vegetable stock or water to a pot large enough to hold them, and bring to a boil. Simmer for 20 to 25 minutes, until the lentils are tender but firm. Drain the liquid and set aside.

You can roast and peel the skin off the bell peppers yourself, but it should be easy to find these already roasted in a jar, which you simply have to drain and chop.

Whisk together all the ingredients for the vinaigrette. Add the bell peppers and chopped herbs to the lentil mix, then fold in the vinaigrette and the crumbled feta.

Add pepper to taste, then serve over 2 to 3 cups of loose mixed salad greens.

Lentil Nut Loaf with Red Pepper Sauce

Contributed by Gail Pettiford Willett
and Walter Willett, MD, DrPH

Lentil Nut Loaf:
1 cup lentils, washed
2 cups water
1 large onion, chopped
1 cup mushrooms, chopped
2 tablespoons olive oil, plus additional oil
  for greasing the baking pan
1 cup walnuts, chopped
1 cup whole wheat breadcrumbs
1 tablespoon lemon juice
1 tablespoon soy sauce
Salt and pepper to taste
1 tablespoon mixed herbs of your choice

Red Pepper Sauce:
2 tablespoons olive oil
3 garlic cloves
1 jar of roasted red pepper
3 tomatoes, chopped
Red pepper flakes (optional)

For lentil loaf: preheat oven to 350 degrees. Grease a baking pan.

Combine lentils and water in a large pot, and cook lentils until they're soft, about half an hour. Heat the olive oil in a sauté pan or skillet, and sauté the onions and mushrooms until they're soft. Mix all other ingredients in with the mushrooms and onions. Sauté for three to four minutes. Place the mixture in the greased baking pan and bake at 350 for 30 minutes.

For red pepper sauce: heat oil in sauté pan or skillet, and sauté the garlic on medium heat for three to four minutes. Add the red pepper and tomatoes. Cook until the mixture thickens— about 15 minutes. Ladle over the lentil loaf. Can be served hot or at room temperature. Makes four servings. (Lentil loaf recipe adapted from Recipes for Natural Health: www.recipes.org/health/main.htm; red pepper sauce recipe adapted from yumyum.com.)

Penne with Broccoli and Sundried Tomatoes
Contributed by Cheryl Greene and Alan Greene, MD

2 ounces (¾ cup) sundried tomatoes,
    julienned
5 cloves garlic, coarsely chopped
¼ cup olive oil
8 ounces whole wheat penne pasta
4 ounces portabella mushrooms, sliced
3 cups fresh broccoli florets, cut into
    bite-sized pieces
4 ounces Kalamata olives or other black olives
4 ounces pasteurized feta cheese
2 ounces Parmesan cheese (optional)

Put the sundried tomatoes and chopped garlic in a small bowl, and pour the olive oil over them. Let stand at least 30 minutes before cooking, or overnight, to allow the tomatoes to reconstitute and the oil to become flavored. If you allow the flavors to marry for longer than four hours, put the bowl in the refrigerator.

Cook the penne according to package directions in a very large cooking pot. While the pasta is cooking, begin cooking the sauce. Heat a large skillet over medium heat, and add the tomato-garlic-oil mixture to the pan. Sauté for one minute. Add the mushrooms and broccoli and sauté over medium heat, stirring occasionally, until the broccoli is tender but still crisp—about five or six minutes.

If the mixture appears dry, add ¼ cup water during the cooking process.

When the pasta is al dente, drain the water and pour the penne back into the cooking pot. Add the tomato, garlic, broccoli, and mushrooms to the pasta. Gently stir in the olives and feta cheese. Mix thoroughly. Sprinkle Parmesan on each serving (if desired). Makes four servings.

Pescado al Cilantro

4 fillets of firm, white-fleshed fish, such
   as flounder, tilapia, cod or haddock
⅔ cup cilantro leaves, rinsed
   and de-stemmed
2 cloves garlic, peeled and chopped
6 tablespoons pickled jalapeño peppers,
   with the juice (about ⅔ of a 7-ounce can)
Black pepper to taste
Lemon wedges and cilantro for garnish

Preheat the broiler. Put the cilantro leaves, garlic, and pickled jalapeños with their juice into a blender. Process them into a paste.

Place the fish onto a broiler pan and spread the blended sauce over the fillets. Grind black pepper over them. Broil for 5 to 10 minutes, depending on the thickness of the fillets, until just cooked through. Sprinkle additional cilantro leaves over cooked fillets for garnish, and serve with cut lemon wedges. Makes four servings.

This recipe is in the Mexican style, but simpler than the traditional method. The sauce is spicy, and the jalapeños are salty, so there's no need to add salt during preparation.

Poached Eggs and Asparagus

1 large bunch asparagus, washed and dried
1 tablespoon grape seed or olive oil
⅓ cup chopped pecans
Four eggs
1 teaspoon white vinegar
¼ cup Parmesan, sliced thin (optional)
1 teaspoon crushed hot pepper flakes (optional)
Pinch salt and freshly ground black and white pepper

To prepare the asparagus: break the ends off each stalk and throw them away. Bring a large pot of water to boil. While waiting for the water to boil, heat the oil in a skillet or sauté pan over medium-high heat. When it's hot but not smoking, add the pecans and a pinch of salt and pepper, stirring often.

When the water boils, blanch the asparagus stalks in it for two to three minutes. Then remove them from the water with a pasta spoon or small colander and transfer to the skillet with the pecans, stirring often. Adjust salt and pepper to taste.

To prepare the eggs: in the same pot of water in which you blanched the asparagus, turn the heat down until the water is at a simmer, and the vinegar. Break one of the eggs into a small bowl, and slide it into the water. Repeat with each of the eggs. With the water at a simmer, let the eggs cook until the whites are just opaque. Then remove each from the water with a slotted spoon and place on a paper towel to drain.

When the asparagus is al dente, serve it and the sautéed pecans on two plates, then top each serving with two poached eggs, several slices of Parmesan for garnish, and a sprinkling of black and white pepper and crushed hot pepper flakes, if desired. Makes two servings.

Pork & Pineapple Curry with Coconut Chutney

Coconut Chutney:

⅔ cup grated coconut (fresh is best,
   if available; if using sweetened prepared
   coconut, do not include sugar or sugar substitute)

1 teaspoon sugar or sugar substitute

⅓ cup low-fat Greek yogurt

1 jalapeño, de-seeded, de-ribbed, and diced

2 tablespoons hot water

1 tablespoon extra-virgin olive oil

1 teaspoon salt

1 teaspoon freshly grated lemon zest

1 teaspoon lemon juice

Pork & Pineapple Curry:

2 12-ounce cans of unsweetened coconut milk

2 tablespoons red curry paste

1 tablespoon curry powder

½ cup low-sodium chicken broth

½ cup water

2 tablespoons fish sauce

1 tablespoon sugar or sugar substitute

1 tablespoon grated ginger

1 cup pineapple, cut into chunks

1 red or yellow pepper, sliced

6 Kaffir lime leaves (optional)

¾ pound lean pork, cut into chunks

½ cup fresh Thai basil (regular basil also works well)

To prepare chutney: puree all ingredients in a blender or food processor. (Can be done ahead and refrigerated for up to two days. Remove from refrigerator for 15 minutes before serving.)

To prepare curry: pour most of the contents of one of the cans of coconut milk into a medium-sized sauté pan or skillet, and heat over medium-high heat for several minutes, stirring regularly, until the coconut milk has thickened. Add the curry paste and curry powder, stirring until both have dissolved (about one minute).

Add the pork, and stir for one or two minutes, until the pork is coated with sauce. Add the remaining coconut milk, chicken broth, water, fish sauce, sugar or sugar substitute, grated ginger, and lime leaves, and bring to a boil.

Reduce heat to a simmer, stirring occasionally, for the next eight or so minutes, until the pork is nearly cooked. Add the pineapple, bell pepper, and basil leaves, and cook for an additional four or five minutes, until the pineapple is soft and the pork is done. Garnish with basil. Serve with about ¼ cup coconut chutney on the side. Makes two servings.

Quinoa & Radish Salad

Contributed by Sophie Barrett and Susannah Smith

1 ½ cups quinoa
3 cups water
1 large or 2 small bell peppers, diced finely
5 radishes, quartered lengthwise and thinly sliced
1 bunch scallions, chopped
¾ cup toasted sliced almonds
½ cup cilantro, chopped
½ cup chiffonade basil
⅓ cup olive oil
The juice of 2 to 2 ½ limes
Salt and freshly ground black pepper

Rinse the quinoa well. In a large pot, bring the quinoa, water, and a pinch of salt to a boil, then reduce the heat to a simmer. Cover the pot, and cook the quinoa until the water has been absorbed and the quinoa is a nice consistency when tested (about 15 to 20 minutes). Remove from the heat and let cool.

In a large serving bowl, mix the cooked quinoa together with the remaining ingredients. Makes four servings.

Salmon with Fava Bean & Spring Pea Mash

Mash:
2 pounds fresh fava beans, in their pods and
   shelled, or 1 pound dried fava beans
1 pound shelled peas
2 cloves garlic, minced or pressed
Zest from half a lemon
2 tablespoons extra-virgin olive oil
2 tablespoons grated Parmesan (optional)
1 teaspoon crushed hot pepper flakes (optional)
Pinch salt and freshly ground black pepper

Salmon:
1 fillet, about ¾ pound
1 tablespoon extra-virgin olive oil
Pinch salt and freshly ground black pepper
Lemon wedges for garnish

To prepare mash if using fresh fava beans: Bring a large pot of water to boil and blanch the fava beans for about two minutes. Scoop them out of the water and deposit them in an ice bath. When they're cool, pinch off their skins. Bring the water on the stove back to a boil and add salt. Put the now-skinned beans back into the boiling water along with the shelled peas, and cook until the favas are very tender. Rinse and drain the favas and peas.

If using dried fava beans: Soak them in cold water overnight. Drain them and remove their skins. (Slicing them with a knife makes this a bit easier.) Put them in a large pot of water over high heat and bring them to a boil. Skim the foam from the water occasionally, and cook the beans for an hour to an hour and a half, or until very tender, stirring often. Add the peas to the water for the last several minutes. Drain the beans and peas.

Heat one tablespoon of the olive oil in a large saucepan and sauté the garlic. Add the fava beans and peas, lemon zest, hot pepper flakes, salt, and pepper. Cook for several minutes over medium heat, adding water as necessary, and stirring often. Using a potato masher, mash the beans to a fairly coarse pulp and fold in the remaining tablespoon of olive oil and the Parmesan. Check the seasoning and adjust salt and pepper as necessary.

To prepare the fish: preheat the broiler. Line the broiling pan with aluminum foil, and coat the foil with a bit of olive oil. Brush the remaining oil over the fish, and sprinkle with salt and pepper. Broil for about six or seven minutes. Cover the fish with aluminum foil and broil for another five or six minutes, or until just cooked through. (This will vary depending on the thickness of the fish.)

On each plate, place about half a cup of mash and top with half of the fish fillet. Garnish with lemon wedges. Makes two servings with plenty of leftover mash.

Spicy Fresh Tuna Salad

Contributed by Eric C. Westman, MD, MHS

2 tablespoons grated lemon zest

2 teaspoons salt

2 teaspoons ground coriander

1 ½ teaspoons freshly ground black pepper

1 ½ teaspoons ground ginger

½ teaspoon ground cumin

3 tablespoons olive oil, divided

4 One-inch thick tuna steaks (about 1 ½ pounds)

2 cups watercress or other salad greens

2 teaspoons balsamic vinegar

1 tablespoon extra-virgin olive oil

Salt and freshly ground black pepper

In a small bowl, combine zest, salt, coriander, pepper, ginger, and cumin. Stir in two tablespoons oil. Rub mixture onto tuna steaks.

Heat remaining tablespoon of oil in a large skillet over high heat until it shimmers. Add steaks and sauté until just cooked through, about four to six minutes, turning halfway through cooking time.

Meanwhile, place vinegar in a small bowl. Slowly whisk in olive oil until dressing slightly thickens. Season to taste with salt and pepper and toss greens with dressing.

Cut fish into ¼-inch slices and serve over greens. Makes four servings.

Spring Straciatella Soup

3 cups unsalted chicken broth
(homemade if you have it)
5 ounces (roughly ½ cup)
cooked chicken, cut up
2 teaspoons salt
1 teaspoon freshly ground black paper
½ cup chopped parsley, preferably Italian
¼ cup grated Parmesan
1 clove fresh green garlic, minced
(optional, but very good)
1 egg

Place the chicken and broth in a large soup pot and heat over medium heat. Add salt and pepper. When the soup comes to a simmer, add the parsley and garlic. Just before serving, whisk in the cheese and the egg. Makes two servings.

··· SIDE DISHES ···

Coleslaw with Mint

Coleslaw:
½ head red cabbage, chopped finely
¼ cup onion (red or sweet), chopped finely
1 green bell pepper, de-ribbed and chopped
1 tablespoon fresh mint leaves, chopped finely

Dressing:
2 tablespoons Dijon mustard
¼ teaspoon salt and fresh-ground pepper to taste
4 drops Tabasco sauce
⅓ cup apple cider vinegar
¼ cup olive oil

Mix together all ingredients for the slaw and set aside.

To make the dressing: whisk ingredients together in a bowl, or pour into a large jar, close the lid tightly, and shake until well blended.

Pour the dressing over the slaw and mix well. Makes four servings.

Curried Sweet Potato Fries

2 pounds sweet potatoes
2 tablespoons olive oil
1 tablespoon curry powder
1 teaspoon cayenne powder (optional)
1 tablespoon salt
Freshly ground black pepper

Preheat the oven to 450 degrees. Peel the sweet potatoes, and cut into ¼- to ½-inch slices, then cut again into ¼- to ½-inch wide strips. Toss the sweet potato pieces and the oil in a large bowl until the pieces are coated. Then mix in the other ingredients and toss. (Be careful with the curry powder: because of the turmeric in it, it will dye everything it touches yellow.)

Line two baking sheets with parchment paper, and spread the potato pieces over them in a single layer. Bake until tender and golden brown, roughly 20 to 30 minutes, turning them occasionally. Makes six servings.

Farmer's Market Saag

3 bunches of fresh greens (we like mixing and
  matching the following, depending on what's
  in season: collards; kale; chard; beet, mustard,
  or turnip greens; spinach; arugula)
The turnips or beets that came with the bunch
  of greens, or two sweet potatoes
1½ tablespoons safflower or grape seed oil
1 teaspoon cumin seeds
2 cloves garlic, pressed or finely minced
1 fresh jalapeño, seeded and minced
  (optional—but good)
1 teaspoon finely minced ginger,
  or ½ teaspoon ginger powder
1 teaspoon Kosher salt
1 ¼ cups boiling water
1 teaspoon garam masala

Wash the greens thoroughly until they have no more grit. Pick through them to remove any yellow or wilted ones. Spin or shake the water out and chop coarsely.

Scrub turnips or beets and cut off tops and tails. If using sweet potatoes, pare off skins. Cut whichever root vegetable you're using into two-inch pieces.

Heat the oil in a large frying pan. (Cast iron works very well.) When the oil is hot, add the cumin seeds and stir until they darken (just a few seconds). Then stir in the garlic and jalapeño, if you're using it. Add your root vegetable pieces and sauté for 6 to 10 minutes, regulating the heat so they don't burn.

Add a handful of the chopped greens and stir them in. When they wilt (which should take less than a minute), add more greens. Keep this up until all the greens are in the pan. Sprinkle them with the ginger and salt, and stir well. Add the boiling water, reduce the heat, and cover the pan. Cook for about 20 additional minutes, or until the root vegetables are tender.

Uncover and cook a bit more, until any excess moisture evaporates. Stir in the garam masala and remove the saag from heat. Makes four servings.

Fennel Salad

1 fennel bulb
2 tablespoons fresh grated Parmesan
1 tablespoon olive oil
1 teaspoon lemon juice
Salt and pepper to taste

To prepare the fennel: Slice off both ends, chop lengthwise, and then cut into thin pieces—an eighth- to a quarter-inch thick in size. Set pieces aside.

To make the dressing: Whisk olive oil, lemon juice, salt and pepper together in your serving bowl with a fork.

Once the dressing is blended, add the fennel and grated cheese and toss. Makes two servings.

Grilled Garlic Green Beans
Contributed by Cheryl Greene and Alan Greene, MD

1½ pounds green beans, washed and trimmed
1½ teaspoons olive oil
½ teaspoon garlic powder
Kosher salt and freshly ground pepper, to taste

In a large bowl, drizzle the olive oil over the green beans. Toss with the garlic powder to distribute evenly.

Heat a grill, grill pan, or cast iron griddle over high heat. Arrange the beans in one layer (you may have to do two batches) and cook without turning until hot all the way through, but still crisp, about three to four minutes. Gently turn the beans over and cook for another three to four minutes, stirring occasionally.

Season with salt and pepper and serve immediately. Makes four servings.

Kale Chips

1 bunch kale, washed, dried, stems and
center ribs removed, and torn into half-inch pieces
1 tablespoon olive oil
Pinch Kosher salt and freshly ground black pepper

Preheat the oven to 300 degrees.

In a large bowl, toss the kale with the olive oil, salt, and pepper. Arrange in a single layer on a baking sheet, and bake until crisp (about 25 to 30 minutes for flat kale, and 30 to 35 for curly).

Let cool on a rack and enjoy. Makes three to four servings.

Naked Salad

Contributed by Cheryl Greene and Alan Greene, MD

1 very ripe avocado, small diced
5 ounces salad greens, washed and spun dry
½ red bell pepper, diced
½ small sweet red onion, thinly sliced
1 small basket (1 dry pint) cherry or grape tomatoes
¾ cup toasted walnuts
1 tablespoon grated Parmesan cheese
Freshly ground pepper, to taste

Combine avocado, salad greens, red pepper, red onion, and tomatoes in an extra-large bowl. Toss the salad liberally so that the avocado breaks down and lightly coats all the vegetables. You shouldn't be able to pick out any avocado pieces when you're done tossing. Pour into serving bowls and top with toasted walnuts, Parmesan cheese, and fresh ground black pepper. Makes four servings.

Roasted Brussels Sprouts

1 pound brussels sprouts
2 tablespoons grape seed or extra-virgin olive oil
½ cup chopped pecans
Pinch salt and freshly ground black pepper
1 teaspoon sugar or sugar substitute (optional)
1 teaspoon balsamic vinegar

Preheat the oven to 400 degrees. While the oven is heating, wash and dry the brussels sprouts, cut off their ends, and halve or quarter them, depending on their size. (The smaller the pieces, the more delicious and tender they will be.)

In a large skillet, heat the oil over medium-high heat until it's hot but not smoking, and add the pecans, salt, and pepper, stirring often to coat the pecan pieces. After several minutes, add the brussels sprouts, along with another sprinkling of salt and pepper.

Turn the burner to medium-low. Stirring occasionally, let the sprouts cook until they start to brown, about eight or nine minutes. Then deglaze the pan with the vinegar, add the sugar or sugar substitute if desired, and stir until the liquid has evaporated (another minute or two more).

Transfer the skillet to the oven and roast until brussels sprouts are tender when pierced with a knife (about three to five additional minutes). Makes four servings.

Roasted Garlic

Contributed by Michael D. Ozner, MD, FACC, FAHA,
author of The Miami Mediterranean Diet, *from which this recipe is taken.*

1 jumbo garlic head
1 hardy pinch of garlic powder
    or garlic salt (optional)
Olive oil to drizzle

Set oven to 400 degrees. Remove only loose leaves from the garlic bulb. Holding the head firmly with stem up, cut off the pointy tops of each clove. Try to keep the remaining leaves and cloves intact.

Place head (stem and cut cloves facing up) in a tight-fitting baking dish. Sprinkle the top of the head with garlic powder or garlic salt, if desired, and drizzle with olive oil. Place in the oven and bake until the head is golden brown on top and the clove tops can be easily pierced with a fork tip. About 20-30 minutes depending on your oven.

Dr. Ozner suggests: "Goes great with pieces of a crusty whole wheat bread or toasted whole wheat pita wedges and a glass of red wine."

Tangy Tangerine Cress Salad

Contributed by Michael D. Ozner, MD, FACC, FAHA,
author of The Miami Mediterranean Diet, *from which this recipe is taken.*

4 large sweet tangerines
Juice from 1 fresh lemon
¼ cup extra virgin olive oil
Sea salt and freshly ground pepper to taste
2 large bunches watercress
   (washed and tough stems removed)
10 cherry tomatoes, halved
16 pitted Kalamata olives

Peel tangerines and separate sections. Remove any pits and squeeze sections to get ¼ cup of juice. Set sections aside.

In a large bowl, whisk together tangerine juice, lemon juice, oil, salt and pepper to taste. Pat watercress dry with paper towels to remove any excess water. Add watercress, tomatoes, and olives to tangerine sections and toss with oil mixture. Serve immediately on chilled salad plates. Makes four servings.

Veggie Dips
Contributed by Cheryl Greene and Alan Greene, MD

Baba Ganoush
1 large eggplant (about 1 ½ pounds)
¾ teaspoon salt
2 cloves garlic
¼ cup lemon juice
2 tablespoons tahini
1 tablespoon extra virgin olive oil
½ teaspoon ground cumin
Kosher salt, to taste

Preheat the oven to 400 degrees. Prick the eggplant with a fork, place it on a cookie sheet, and roast for about 40 minutes or until very soft inside. Allow to cool completely.

Scoop out the eggplant's pulp and process in a food processor with the remaining ingredients until it is almost pureed but still has some texture. Adjust seasoning to taste.

Refrigerate until ready to use. Makes 1 ½ cups of baba ganoush.

Hummus
2 cups dried garbanzo beans (chickpeas)
½ cup lemon juice (4-5 lemons)
½ teaspoon salt
⅓ to ½ cup water
⅓ cup extra virgin olive oil
½ cup tahini

Soak the dried garbanzo beans in a large bowl with 6 cups of water for at least 3 hours or overnight. Drain, transfer to a medium sauce-pan, and cover with cold water to at least 2 inches above the level of the beans. Bring to a boil, and then cook gently over medium heat until very soft, about 45 minutes.

Drain the beans and pulse in a food processer with the lemon juice, salt, and 1/3 cup water until very smooth. Add the olive oil and tahini, and process again until completely smooth and creamy. If the hummus is too thick, add a bit more water. Makes four cups.

The Greenes say: "These Mediterranean-inspired veggie dips are great for your toddler, and as dips for lunch, dinner, or a casual party. They make new veggies welcome!"

Wheat Berry Salad

*Contributed by Jeffrey Blumberg, PhD and
Helen Rasmussen, PhD, RD, FADA.*

*The recipe below is based on one used in a clinical trial
created at the Human Nutrition Research Center on Aging.*

1 cup prepared wheat berries
   (see preparation method, below)
½ teaspoon chicken bouillon (cube or loose granules;
   can use low-sodium bouillon)
⅓ cup water
2 tablespoons finely sliced onion
⅛ teaspoon ground black pepper
1 clove garlic, minced or pressed
2 tablespoons lemon juice
½ tablespoon olive oil
1 tablespoon dry wheat bran
2 tablespoons chopped walnuts

To prepare wheat berries: measure one cup of dry berries into a saucepan (or use a rice cooker, if you prefer). Add two and a half cups of water and bring to a boil. Stir the berries, lower the heat to a simmer, and cook for 20 minutes. Check to see that there is still adequate water to prevent scorching. Cook for another 40 minutes, or until the berries are soft.

To prepare salad: dissolve the chicken bouillon in water. In a serving bowl, mix the dissolved bouillon, lemon juice, and olive oil. Stir in onions, pepper, and garlic. Add the cup of cooked wheat berries, wheat bran, and walnuts. Mix together. Makes one serving.

Here is Dr. Blumberg and Dr. Rasmussen's story of how this recipe came to be:

> "This salad was created for use in a study to compare diets containing low versus high glycemic index foods. The glycemic index ranks dietary carbohydrates from 1 to 100 according to their ability to increase blood glucose (sugar) concentrations. Foods with a lower glycemic index produce smaller increases in blood glucose and insulin than those with a high glycemic index.
>
> "The glycemic load is a calculation of the glycemic index and the portion size; servings of foods with a high glycemic load have values of 20 and higher. This wheat berry salad has a low glycemic index and glycemic load (45 and 10, respectively). Foods with a high glycemic index or glycemic load have been associated with a greater risk for diabetes."

··· DESSERTS ···

Blueberry Cheesecake
Contributed by Steven Zeisel, MD, PhD
and Susan Zeisel, Ed.D.

1 pint blueberries
1 tablespoon cornstarch
1 pound reduced-fat cream cheese
   at room temperature
1 pound fat-free cream cheese at
   room temperature
Finely grated rind of 1 lemon
3 tablespoons lemon juice
2 teaspoons vanilla extract
1½ cups sugar
2 eggs
½ cup egg substitute such as Egg Beaters

Preheat oven to 350 degrees. Grease an eight-inch cheesecake pan (it does not have a loose bottom and is about three inches high). Be sure to grease entire pan or cake will stick.

Purée blueberries in a blender with the cornstarch. Pour mixture into a small saucepan and heat for about five minutes or until thickened. Set aside.

Mix both pounds of cream cheese in a mixer until smooth. Scrape down the sides of the bowl. Add the sugar and beat. Add the lemon juice, vanilla, and lemon rind and beat. Add the eggs, one at a time, beating until just combined. Then beat in the egg substitute.

Pour the cream cheese mixture into the greased pan. Smooth top. Spread blueberry purée over the top. Using a knife, swirl the purée through the cheese mixture to marble.

Place the pan into a larger pan that is filled with one inch of water. Bake for one and a half hours. (The top of the cake should be dry, but the inside should be soft.)

Remove the cake pan from the larger pan and place on a rack. Allow the cake pan to cool until the bottom reaches room temperature. When cool, carefully turn the pan over a flat board. Carefully re-invert onto a cake plate. Do not press too hard or you will squash the cake. Refrigerate for five to six hours or freeze. Serve cold. Makes eight servings.

Cantaloupe with Lime & Mint

One ripe cantaloupe, cut into large chunks
1 tablespoon of fresh lime juice
¼ cup fresh mint (chiffonade)

Pour the lime juice over the cantaloupe and allow to sit for one or two minutes. Garnish with the mint chiffonade and serve in dessert bowls. Makes four servings.

Fresh Fruit Kabobs and Cinnamon Honey Dip
Contributed by Michael D. Ozner, MD, FACC, FAHA,
author of The Miami Mediterranean Diet, *from which this recipe is taken.*

Assorted seasonal fresh fruit, cut into chunks
  (enough for four 8-inch wooden skewers)
2 cups low-fat plain yogurt, well chilled
4 tablespoons honey
Pinch of ground white pepper
6-8 teaspoons ground cinnamon, or to taste
A non-caloric sweetener to taste, if desired
Extra ground cinnamon to sprinkle

Prepare assorted fruits on skewers. Combine yogurt, honey, pepper, cinnamon, and sweetener in a large bowl and stir to blend. Serve each kabob on a plate drizzled with ¼ of yogurt mixture and sprinkled with a small amount of ground cinnamon. Serves four.

Key Lime Custard

1 14-ounce can of sweetened condensed milk
6 egg yolks
½ cup fresh-squeezed key lime juice
2-3 crushed ginger snaps
2 tablespoons crystallized ginger, diced small
4 tablespoons fresh berries (raspberries or blueberries work well)

Preheat the oven to 375 degrees. In a medium-sized bowl, whisk together the condensed milk and egg yolks. Then, very slowly, stir in the key lime juice. It will cause the milk to curdle and then thicken, so it should only be added a little at a time, and you should whisk constantly.

Pour the mixture into four ramekins (the mixture will rise slightly during baking, so leave a bit of room). Place the ramekins inside a large baking pan that has one inch of water in the bottom of it, and then place the baking pan on a baking sheet. Slide the baking sheet onto a center rack in the oven.

Bake until the custard is set, about 15 minutes. Remove from the oven and place on a cooling rack. Once at room temperature, cover each ramekin in saran, and refrigerate for at least several hours or up to a couple of days before serving.

Garnish each serving with ginger snap crumbs, caramelized ginger, and one tablespoon of berries. Serves four.

Poached Pears with Bittersweet Cocoa Sauce

Contributed by Teresa Graedon, PhD and Kit Gruelle,
co-authors of Chocolate Without Guilt, *from which this recipe is taken.*

Pears:
2 pears, ripe but firm
4 tablespoons raspberries (can substitute frozen)
4 tablespoons bittersweet cocoa sauce (see below)
1 cup water
2 tablespoons sugar
1½ cups white wine
1 cup orange juice
Strip orange zest

Cocoa Sauce:
¾ cup cocoa
¾ cup sugar
¾ cup water
½ cup skim milk
1 tablespoon vanilla extract
3 tablespoons nonfat yogurt
pinch salt (optional)

To prepare the cocoa sauce: Combine sugar and cocoa (and salt if desired) in a saucepan and mix together. Add the water and mix with a wire whisk until well blended and smooth. (Mixture will be quite thick.) Place over medium-low heat and stir constantly until it is well heated and the sugar has dissolved completely. Add the vanilla extract, stir in the milk and yogurt, and blend thoroughly. Serve warm. (Makes 18 servings of 2 tablespoons each.)

To make the poaching syrup: Combine the water, orange juice, wine, orange zest, and sugar in a small heavy saucepan and put it over medium heat. Stir it for just a minute, then let it simmer slowly until the sugar dissolves.

In the meantime, halve the pears, then core and peel them. Immediately drop them into the simmering syrup and cook them gently for about 20 minutes. (Smaller or riper pears may need a few minutes less; larger or firmer pears may need 5 or so minutes more.) This step is important, so be careful with the pears while they are poaching. They need to stay firm rather than become mushy and fall apart, which may happen if they are overcooked. Since you don't want to have to start over, test them often by poking gently with a sharp knife.

When the pears are tender enough to be pierced easily, take them out of the poaching liquid with a slotted spoon and allow them to cool to room temperature.

When the pears have cooled, place each half on a dessert plate, hollow side up. Fill the hollow of each one with about a tablespoon of raspberries and then drizzle a tablespoon of cocoa syrup over the berries. Makes four servings.

Roasted Peaches

    3 firm but ripe peaches, de-fuzzed, halved, and pitted
    1 teaspoon butter
    ¼ cup sliced almonds, toasted
    3 tablespoons honey
    2½ cups low-fat Greek yogurt

Preheat the oven to 350 degrees. Grease a glass baking dish with the butter, and arrange the peaches in it, sliced side up. Roast until peaches are tender when pierced with the tip of a sharp knife (about 30 to 35 minutes).

Serve one peach half with ½ cup yogurt. Top each serving with about half a tablespoon of honey and a sprinkling of toasted almonds. Makes six servings.

Three-Layer Mousse

Contributed by Teresa Graedon, PhD and Kit Gruelle,
co-authors of Chocolate Without Guilt, *from which this recipe is taken.*

Chocolate Layer:
⅔ cup cocoa
¾ cup sugar
¾ cup skim milk
1 egg yolk
1 package (2 tablespoons) unflavored gelatin
¼ cup cold water
5 egg whites
3 tablespoons sugar
1 cup fromage blanc

Raspberry Layer:
20 ounces frozen unsweetened raspberries
½ cup sugar
1 package unflavored gelatin
¼ cup cold water
4 tablespoons kirsch
3 egg whites
½ cup lowfat silken tofu (like Mori-Nu Lite)
2 tablespoons sugar

Pear Layer:
3 or 4 nearly ripe pears (about 2 pounds)
2 tablespoons water
¼ cup sugar
1 tablespoon Cointreau or Grand Marnier
1 package unflavored gelatin
¼ cup cold water
½ cup lowfat silken tofu
3 egg whites
2 tablespoons sugar

To prepare the chocolate layer: Sprinkle the gelatin on the cold water to soften for five minutes. Meanwhile, in a small saucepan, blend the cocoa, sugar, and milk. Cook it slowly over low heat, stirring constantly until the sugar has dissolved. Beat in the egg yolk, remove the custard from the heat, and allow it to cool. Warm the gelatin and water over low heat, stirring until the gelatin has completely dissolved and the mixture is clear. Add it to the chocolate mixture, then stir in the fromage blanc until it is thoroughly mixed.

Beat the egg whites in a mixer until they are foamy. Gradually add the sugar, still beating, until the peaks are firm but not dry. Gently fold the beaten egg white into the chocolate mixture and spoon it into 12 small glass parfait cups or dessert bowls. Refrigerate while making additional layers.

To prepare the raspberry layer: Sprinkle the gelatin on the cold water to soften for five minutes. Purée the partially thawed raspberries in a food processor along with the ½ cup sugar, kirsch, and tofu. Warm the gelatin and water in a small saucepan over low heat, stirring until the gelatin has completely dissolved and the mixture is clear. With the processor running, pour in the gelatin solution and process thoroughly.

In a clean mixer bowl with clean beaters, beat the egg whites until they are foamy. Add the 2 tablespoons of sugar gradually and continue beating until the peaks are stiff and shiny. Fold the beaten egg whites into the raspberry mixture, and spoon into the serving dishes over the chocolate layer. Refrigerate while making the pear layer.

To prepare the pear layer: Peel, quarter and core the pears. Cut them into slices and put them into a heavy stainless steel or enamel saucepan. Add the 2 tablespoons of water and cook the pear pieces over low heat until they are heated through, about 7 to 10 minutes. Drain off the liquid and put the pears into the food processor.

Soften the gelatin in ¼ cup cold water while you process the pears with the ¼ cup sugar until the mixture is very smooth and the sugar has dissolved. Warm the gelatin and water in a small saucepan over low heat, stirring until the gelatin has completely dissolved and the mixture is clear. With the processor running, pour in the gelatin solution and process thoroughly. Then add the liqueur and the tofu, and process again until the mixture is entirely smooth. The mixture should be at room temperature.

In a clean mixer bowl with clean beaters, beat the egg whites until they are foamy. Add the remaining sugar and continue beating until the egg whites are shiny and stiff. Gently fold the egg whites into the pear mixture and spoon over the raspberry layer. Place the serving dishes in the freezer and freeze for three hours or so. This can be done ahead and frozen overnight. Makes 12 servings.

We recommend putting this dessert into glass serving bowls because it is so beautiful to see the three layers: pale yellow pear, bright pink raspberry, and dark brown chocolate. It is one of our very favorites for the blend of flavors as well. The liqueurs add to the flavor, but they could be eliminated. Fromage blanc is a nonfat soft cheese product that can be found in many health food stores. If it is not available, substitute nonfat ricotta cheese.

HEALTH NOTE: This recipe calls for uncooked egg whites. To avoid salmonella, use pasteurized eggs or reconstitute a powdered egg-white product such as Just Whites.

··· CONTRIBUTORS ···

SOPHIE BARRETT has 10 years of experience working in the food and wine business in both North Carolina and New York. Currently a sales person at Chambers Street Wines in lower Manhattan, she spends her free evenings preparing fresh and healthy food based on seasonal ingredients.

JEFFREY BLUMBERG, PhD, is a Professor in the Friedman School of Nutrition Science and Policy and Director of the Antioxidants Research Laboratory at the Jean Mayer USDA Human Nutrition Research Center on Aging at Tufts University. His research efforts are focused on the biochemical basis for the role of antioxidant nutrients and their dietary requirements in health promotion and disease prevention during the aging process via their modulation of oxidative stress status. He has served on committees of the FDA, WHO, FAO/UN, U.S. Surgeon General's Office, and U.S. Olympic Committee.

CHRISTOPHER GARDNER has a PhD in Nutrition Science from UC Berkeley and is currently an Associate Professor of Medicine at Stanford University. He has been a vegetarian for 27 years, as are his four sons, ages

2, 4, 16, and 19 (his wife is a near-vegetarian/flexitarian). In his research, he has studied the potential health benefits of plant-based diets, garlic, soy, omega-3 fats, and weight-loss diets, among others. His current research passion is studying and advancing the growing social movement around food-related issues. Interests include fatherhood, husbandhood, rock-climbing, volleyball, lacrosse, ultimate frisbee, guitar, calligraphy, composting, and home vegetable gardening.

ALAN GREENE, MD, is President and CEO of DrGreene.com, a Clinical Professor of Pediatrics at Stanford University School of Medicine, an Attending Physician at Packard Children's Hospital, the Founding President and Co-Chair of the Society for Participatory Medicine, and on the board of directors of Healthy Child Healthy World and the Organic Center. He is the Deputy Editor of the *Journal of Participatory Medicine* and the author of many popular health and parenting books including *Raising Baby Green* and *Feeding Baby Green*. He has been featured in the New York Times and has appeared on CNN, *The TODAY Show*, *Good Morning America Health*, NBC *Evening News*, *World News Tonight with Diane Sawyer*, and *The Dr. Oz Show*. Dr. Greene was honored as one of "the 100 most creative and influential innovators working in health care today" and was named the Children's Health Hero of the Internet by Intel.

CHERYL GREENE is the Co-founder and Executive Producer of DrGreene. com, a pediatric web site founded in 1995. She is also a Senior Fellow at the University of California San Francisco, Center for the Health Professions. She is on the board of directors of the Society for Participatory Medicine and X2HN (Women Healthcare Executives Network) and is a supporter of Vitamin Angels. She is a "foodie" and enjoys dishes from different cultures. Her recipes take advantage of whole foods, healthy oils, fiber rich ingredients, and a variety of spices.

KIT GRUELLE has been an advocate for battered women and their children for more than 25 years. She is a domestic violence and sexual assault Subject Matter Expert and trains advocates, criminal justice, and health care professionals across the country. She is finishing a documentary on the American battered women's movement: *Private Violence*. Kit is also an amateur pastry chef with a special love for all things chocolate. She co-authored *Chocolate Without Guilt* (2002) with Terry Graedon. She lives in the Boone, NC area and has three children and two grandchildren.

MARK LIPONIS, MD, has been a practicing clinician in internal medicine for 20 years, and has also had many years of experience in emergency departments and critical care units. He has always had an interest in holistic approaches to health, and began a wellness program as an adjunct to his private practice in Montana in the late eighties. He has continued to expand his understanding and expertise in integrative medicine through his work at Canyon Ranch (www.canyonranch.com). He became Corporate Medical Director of Canyon Ranch in 2003, overseeing medical programming at all Canyon Ranch properties. Dr. Liponis is also the author of two books: *Ultraprevention* (2005), a New York Times bestseller; and *UltraLongevity* published by Little Brown (2007). Dr. Liponis is a national speaker, and has appeared on a number of national television segments on health and wellness, including *The Rachel Ray Show*, CNN, *The TODAY Show*, *The Jane Pauley Show*, and *The View*. He is also a contributing editor to *Parade* and *Healthy Styles* magazines.

TIERAONA LOW DOG, MD, is Clinical Associate Professor and Director of the Fellowship for the Arizona Center for Integrative Medicine at the University of Arizona. Dr. Low Dog was appointed to the White House Commission on Complementary and Alternative Medicine by President Clinton, and she was elected Chair of the United States Pharmacopeia Dietary Supplements—Botanicals Expert Committee from 2000–2010. She is also the recipient of the 2010 People's Pharmacy Award.

His holistic approach to health led DAVID MATHIS, MD, FAAFP, ABHM, D.Ay. to study Ayurveda in both the U.S. and India, becoming the first board-certified family physician to combine Ayurveda and family medicine. Former head of family medicine at Inova Loudoun Hospital Center, he holds an Associate Professorship of Primary Care Medicine at George Washington University School of Medicine, a CCHP in

Correctional Medicine, and has advanced training in infectious diseases. Dr. Mathis lectures frequently on Ayurvedic topics and maintains a private Ayurvedic medical practice.

After Ayurvedic studies in Boston, Albuquerque, and India, DEBBIE MATHIS, MA, D.Ay. joined her husband in their pioneering Integrative Medicine practice and directed its Panchakarma program. She also established ayurveda-md.com, a website introducing Ayurveda's health wisdom to the public. Debbie recently created a jewelry line based on Ayurvedic gem therapy principles, continues to develop and administer Ayurvedic workshops for a variety of audiences, and assists Dr. Mathis with patient consultations.

SALLY FALLON MORELL is founding president of the Weston A. Price Foundation and author of the bestselling *Nourishing Traditions: The Cookbook that Challenges Politically Correct Nutrition and the Diet Dictocrats.*

MICHAEL OZNER, MD, FACC, FAHA, is one of America's leading advocates for heart disease prevention and a well known regional and national speaker in the field of preventive cardiology. He has been featured in the major print, radio, and television media including the *New York Times*, NPR radio, and CBS *News*. Dr. Ozner is a board certified cardiologist, a Fellow of the American College of Cardiology and American Heart Association, Medical Director of Wellness & Prevention at Baptist Health South Florida, and past Chairman of the American Heart Association of Miami. Dr. Ozner is author of *The Miami Mediterranean Diet* and *The Great American Heart Hoax*. For further information: www.drozner.com.

HELEN RASMUSSEN, PhD, RD, FADA, is the Senior Clinical Research Dietitian at the Jean Mayer, USDA Human Nutrition Research Center on Aging (HNRCA) at Tufts University, where she helps develop and implement the feeding component of the clinical nutrition research protocols. Helen is an active member of the faculty, teaching graduate students completing their internships at the Friedman School of Nutrition Science and Policy at Tufts. She also serves on the Board of Directors of Community

Servings, a Massachusetts-based organization that serves home-delivered meals to the critically ill.

SUSANNAH SMITH is manager of Chapel Hill's natural wine/coffee shop, 3CUPS, and spends all free moments thinking about food and drink.

ERIC WESTMAN, MD, MHS, is associate professor of medicine at Duke University Health System and director of the Duke Lifestyle Medicine Clinic. Together with Dr. Stephen Phinney and Dr. Jeff Volek, he is the author of *The New Atkins for a New You*.

WALTER C. WILLETT, MD, Dr PH, is Professor of Epidemiology and Nutrition and Chairman of the Department of Nutrition at Harvard School of Public Health and Professor of Medicine at Harvard Medical School. Dr. Willett has focused much of his work over the last 30 years on the development of methods to study the effects of diet on the oc-currence of major diseases. He has applied these methods in the Nurses' Health Studies I and II and the Health Professionals Follow-up Study. Together, these cohorts are providing the most detailed information on the long-term health consequences of food choices. Dr. Willett has pub-lished over 1,200 articles, primarily on lifestyle risk factors for heart dis-ease and cancer, and has written the textbook Nutritional Epidemiology, as well as three books for the general public: *Eat, Drink and Be Healthy: The Harvard Medical School Guide to Healthy Eating*, which has appeared on most major bestseller lists; *Eat, Drink, and Weigh Less*, co-authored with Mollie Katzen; and most recently, *The Fertility Diet*, co-authored with Jorge Chavarro and Pat Skerrett. Dr. Willett is the most cited nu-tritionist internationally, and is among the five most cited persons in all fields of clinical science. He is a member of the Institute of Medicine of the National Academy of Sciences and the recipient of many national and international awards for his research.

GAIL PETTIFORD WILLETT, RN, has worked in the Human Service field for over 30 years and founded Savanna Books, a multicultural chil-dren's bookstore. She travels extensively and is an avid quilter. She en-joys eating and trying new foods. In recent years she has offered cooking classes to introduce people to new ways of incorporating delicious and healthy foods into their diets, focusing on greens, whole grains, and nuts. She lives in Cambridge with her husband. They have two grown sons.

STEVEN ZEISEL, MD, PhD, is Director of the Nutrition Research Institute at the University of North Carolina. He is also the Kenan Distinguished University Professor in the Departments of Nutrition and Pediatrics at the University of North Carolina and Director of the Human Clinical Nutrition Research Center there.

SUSAN ZEISEL, Ed.D, is a researcher at FPG Child Development Institute at the University of North Carolina at Chapel Hill. She is a pediatric nurse practitioner by training and has an interest in child health. Cooking, especially baking, has been a longtime hobby. She has been working at making things healthier and tasty!

··· ABOUT THE AUTHORS···

··· JOE GRAEDON, MS ···

JOE GRAEDON received his BS from Pennsylvania State University in 1967 and then did research on mental illness, sleep, and basic brain physiology at the New Jersey Neuropsychiatric Institute in Princeton. In 1971 he earned his MS in pharmacology from the University of Michigan. Joe was conferred the degree of Doctor of Humane Letters honoris causa from Long Island University in 2006 as one of the country's leading drug experts for the consumer.

Joe has lectured at the Duke University School of Nursing, the University of California, San Francisco (UCSF) School of Pharmacy, and the University of North Carolina School of Pharmacy. From 1971 to 1974 he taught pharmacology at the School of Medicine of the Universidad Autonoma "Benito Juarez" of Oaxaca, Mexico. He served as a consultant to the Federal Trade Commission on over-the-counter drug issues from 1978 to 1983 and was on the Advisory Board for the Drug Studies Unit at UCSF from 1983 to 1989. He has been an adjunct assistant professor, Division of Pharmacy Practice and Experiential Education, UNC Eshelman School of Pharmacy, at Chapel Hill since 1986 and was a member of the National

Policy Advisory Board for the UNC Center for Education and Research on Therapeutics (CERTS). He is a member of the American Association for the Advancement of Science (AAAS), the Society for Neuroscience, and the New York Academy of Science. Joe was elected to the rank of AAAS Fellow for "exceptional contribution to the communication of the rational use of pharmaceutical products and an understanding of health issues to the public" in 2005.

Joe has served as an editorial advisor to *Men's Health Newsletter* and serves as an editorial advisor to *Prevention* magazine. Joe is an advisory board member of the American Botanical Council (Herbalgram) and he has served as a member of the Board of Visitors, UNC Eshelman School of Pharmacy, since 1989. He also serves on the Patient Safety and Clinical Quality Committee of the Duke University Health System Board of Directors.

Joe's features on health and pharmaceuticals have been syndicated nationally to public television stations via Intraregional Program Service member exchange. He co-authored a novel, *No Deadly Drug* (Pocket Books, 1992), with Tom Ferguson, MD. A TV pledge special was underwritten by PBS in 1998. He is considered one of the country's leading drug experts for consumers and speaks frequently on issues of pharmaceuticals, nutrition, herbs, home remedies, and self-care. He has appeared as a guest on many major U.S. national television shows, including *Dateline, 20/20, The Geraldo Rivera Show, The Oprah Winfrey Show, Live with Regis and Kathie Lee, The TODAY Show, Good Morning America,* CBS *Morning News,* NBC *Nightly News with Tom Brokaw, Extra, The Phil Donahue Show,* and *The Tonight Show with Johnny Carson.*

⋯ TERESA GRAEDON, PHD ⋯

Medical anthropologist TERESA GRAEDON is a best-selling author, syndicated newspaper columnist, and award-winning internationally syndicated radio talk-show host. Teresa Graedon graduated magna cum laude with an AB from Bryn Mawr College in 1969, majoring in anthropology. She attended graduate school at the University of Michigan, receiving her AM in 1971. She received a fellowship from the Institute for Environmental Quality (1972–1975), which enabled her to pursue doctoral research on health and nutritional status in a migrant community in Oaxaca, Mexico.

Her doctorate was awarded in 1976.

Teresa taught at the Duke University School of Nursing with an adjunct appointment in the Department of Anthropology from 1975 to 1979. Thereafter she periodically taught courses in medical anthropology and international health at Duke University. From 1982 to 1983 she pursued postdoctoral training in medical anthropology at the University of California, San Francisco. With Kit Gruelle, she co-authored a cookbook, *Chocolate without Guilt* (Graedon Enterprises, 2002).

Teresa is a Fellow of the Society for Applied Anthropology and a member of the American Anthropological Association and the Society for Medical Anthropology. She previously served on the Foundation Board of the University of North Carolina School of Nursing and the Patient Safety and Clinical Quality Committee of the Duke University Health System Board of Directors. She serves as an editorial advisor to *Prevention* magazine.

··· JOE AND TERRY ···

For over a decade Joe and Terry contributed a regular column on self-medication for Tom Ferguson, MD's magazine, *Medical Self-Care*. Their thrice-weekly newspaper column, The People's Pharmacy, has been syndicated nationally by King Features Syndicate since 1978. The People's Pharmacy radio show won a Silver Award from the Corporation for Public Broadcasting in 1992. It is syndicated to hundreds of radio stations in the United States and around the world on public radio, Radio Reading Service stations, and commercial broadcasters HealthStar® and TalkStar® Radio Networks. In 2003 Joe and Teresa received the Alvarez Award at the 63rd annual conference of the American Medical Writers Association for "Excellence in Medical Communications." Joe & Terry were named "Hometown Heroes" through the WCHL Village Pride Award in 2009.

Joe and Terry were charter members of the North Carolina Consortium of Natural Medicine and Public Health and served on the Consortium Executive Committee in 2003. Joe and Terry serve on the Patient Advocacy Council of Duke University Health System.

The Graedons have coauthored the following books: *The People's Pharmacy-2* (Avon, 1980); *Joe Graedon's The New People's Pharmacy: Drug*

Breakthroughs for the '80s (Bantam, 1985); *The People's Pharmacy, Totally New and Revised* (St. Martin's Press, 1985); *50+: The Graedons' People's Pharmacy for Older Adults* (Bantam, 1988); *Graedons' Best Medicine: From Herbal Remedies to High-Tech Rx Breakthroughs* (Bantam, 1991); *The Aspirin Handbook: A User's Guide to the Breakthrough Drug of the '90s* (Bantam, 1993); *The People's Guide to Deadly Drug Interactions* (St. Martin's Press, 1995; 1997); *The People's Pharmacy, Completely New and Revised* (1996, 1998); *The People's Pharmacy Guide to Home and Herbal Remedies* (St. Martin's Press, 1999); *Best Choices from The People's Pharmacy* (Rodale, 2006, 2007); *Favorite Home Remedies from The People's Pharmacy* (Graedon Enterprises, 2008) and *Favorite Foods from The People's Pharmacy: Mother Nature's Medicine* (Graedon Enterprises, 2009).

Total books in print well exceed 2 million. Terry and Joe contributed a chapter on over-the-counter medications to *The Merck Manual of Medical Information Home Edition* (1997) and to *Health Care Choices for Today's Consumer: Guide to Quality and Cost* (1997).

Terry and Joe were presented with the America Talks Health "Health Headliner of 1998" award for "superior contribution to the advancement of medicine and public health education." Together they have been designated Ambassadors Plenipotentiary by the City of Medicine, Durham, North Carolina, where they live. You can communicate with the Graedons through their Web site, www.peoplespharmacy.com, or write to them at:

GRAEDON ENTERPRISES, INC.
P. O. Box 52027
Durham, NC 27717-2027